I0491485

The Double-Edged Sword

Christopher Turnbull

Kindle Direct Publishing, United States of America

Introduction

From a young age, I was well aware of the term paramedic. My father had served in the local volunteer fire company from the 1970s until shortly after my birth. Years later we would attend a pool party in the summer with his old comrades so he could reunite with the guys who always had his back in the most dangerous of conditions. In attendance was a man named John. John was a respected paramedic. I could see that from a young age by his popularity with those in attendance. This guy was a real hero. I knew then that he did something great for so many people. But I had no idea *what* he did.

The Double-Edged Sword

I was born into a Roman Catholic family, attending church every Sunday, trying to sit in the same seat every Sunday, and doing the same worship rituals every Sunday. I grew up in Sunday school learning about and receiving the timely sacraments. When I was in 6th grade, I was moved from public to Catholic school and had served as an Altar boy.

My parents divorced around the same time as this change to schools. During my freshman year of high school, I went to move in with my dad who lived in a small town with very little to do. I finished my freshman year at the Catholic High School then moved back to a public school. I had heard of some of my peers from school being "junior firefighters," so I pursued the activity following in my father's footsteps.

There was a night that I found myself observing an emergency scene from my dad's house across the street from a local grocery store that had a large turnout of fire apparatus. A man was parked on the road waving an orange illuminated baton keeping the flow of traffic moving on a busy-by-day, dead-by-night state road. He was an older, stocky man with a cigar hanging out of his mouth as he stood there in fluorescent yellow attire watching traffic to ensure the safety of the firefighters on the job. I made my way over to him and asked how to become a junior firefighter. Surprisingly it was as easy as stopping by the fire station with my dad anytime somebody was there to do some paperwork.

In August 2001, I responded to my first emergency with the fire department, a motor vehicle collision with injuries. It was overwhelming but awe-inspiring to see how multiple agencies came together on the same location with different goals about the same accident. The police conducted their investigation while the EMTs took the injured parties from the wreckage. The fire department made sure vehicle fluids were contained and cleaned up while also maintaining a safe environment for the EMTs to do their job. I grabbed a bucket of oil drying material and dispensed it onto some fluids following the example of another volunteer from my rescue apparatus. Once the incident was cleared up with the vehicle towed off the intersection, we returned to the firehouse and to our respective homes.

For the first time in my life I was operating side by side with the same sort of people I had spent my entire youth looking up to. I was a member of something bigger than myself. I had a huge sense of pride that would lead every conversation for years to come. From here on out, any time not spent at home was time spent at the firehouse, no more church on Sunday.

I went on to meet a girl within the fire company who later approached me because she wanted to become an EMT. She found a class and didn't have a "partner" to go through it with, so I thought it might be good to attend with her. After all, one day I was going to be a big deal firefighter, so having an EMT certificate in my file would be helpful in my advancement. I finished high school and joined the Army Reserve which suddenly put a halt to my training on weekends, leaving me unable to further my competency within the fire company or as an EMT.

4

Christopher Turnbull

Upon returning home from basic training, I took a job with a non-emergency transportation ambulance company. I spent my days taking people places in a wheelchair or stretcher van to doctors appointments from nursing homes and transferring hospital discharges to rehab facilities. I found a paycheck with the EMT certificate I obtained in high school and met the minimum educational requirements to maintain the associated card that expired every three years. My third year at this employer was interrupted by deployment with the Army. I returned home and immediately returned to my employment duties while picking up shifts at the local volunteer emergency ambulance with little to no guidance. I had a very entry-level foundation that I had not challenged myself to improve upon five years after receiving my initial certification. The transportation company that I was working for was closed, and I was met with a crossroads for the first time in my career.

I took a job offer from the local hospital-based ambulance service. This service's paramedic component covered the vast majority of the county I was working in. At my interview I was

asked to make a decision: I could continue with the type of

transportation I was doing or I could begin training into a spot on

the emergency side of the organization. This would include a

vigorous process of observing senior EMTs in their interactions

with patients, being taught the expectations and protocols, and

learning to drive with the lights and siren activated. After my

orientation period ended, I was able to care for sick and injured

patients with the assistance of the paramedics on critically sick

people.

In this book, I discuss my experiences in the emergency

services noting stressors, victories, pitfalls, relationships, and how

twenty years of service has ultimately brought me to seek Jesus

Christ. The stories shared are my own experiences, with some

names changed to protect the privacy of others. We have a job to

do. It's a job that many members of the general public regard to be

impossible for them to do. Somehow we found our way into this

career where the expectation is that we are saving lives. We give

100% every day in conditions that many others would otherwise run from, quite literally in some situations. We embark on a long career with ups and downs that come at any time from every angle, to every provider.

This book is a sharing of events that have helped shape me into who I am today; a husband, a father, and a confident paramedic. The beginning of my journey from casual Christian towards one of Jesus' disciples is detailed as well. My experience is just one of many providers worldwide and may be vastly different from others with my tenure, or maybe it is similar to experiences another person has struggled with or is going through right now.

Although our individual experiences in EMS might be different, the expectations in this line of work are the same. There is a widely accepted mentality that it is our job to save people. We give constantly then return after shift to manage our home lives just to turn around and do it all again. We give so much of ourselves in a variety of situations. At what point do we realize that we are approaching burnout? What happens when the people

who are expected to make everything better are realizing that they

themselves are not okay? We make a career of trying to save

strangers; but when we need it most, who is there to save us? This

is The Double-Edged "S"word.

<u>Chapter 1: Who Are We?</u>

"A man was going down from Jerusalem to Jericho, when he was attacked by robbers. They stripped him of his clothes, beat him and went away, leaving him half dead. A priest happened to be going down the same road, and when he saw the man, he passed by on the other side. So too, a Levite, when he came to the place and saw him, passed by on the other side. But a Samaritan, as he traveled, came where the man was; and when he saw him, he took pity on him. He went to him and bandaged his wounds, pouring on oil and wine. Then he put the man on his own donkey, brought him

to an inn and took care of him." Luke 10: 30-34.

Isn't it funny how citizens come across a person on the

street and can identify that they need assistance but seldom render

any form of aid besides calling the emergency phone number?

This concept isn't new. It has been in the Bible for generations.

It's easy to walk around somebody in need and not get involved or

to call for help with plenty of distance between you and the other

person. But there are some of us who see the needs and respond to

them whether we are the ones to come across the need or if we are

dispatched to their location.

An Emergency Medical Technician (EMT) is a prehospital

healthcare provider who is trained in basic life support. They are

CPR-certified and proficient in basic emergency care such as

oxygen administration, bandaging, splinting, and also provide a

second set of hands in situations where a paramedic has primary

care. Their assessment is vital in leading a care-centered team

approach to patient care.

Christopher Turnbull
A Paramedic (Medic) is a prehospital healthcare provider who is trained in the same disciplines as EMTs, in addition to advanced life support practices. Medics are given a variety of medications and protocols and coordinate with doctors at receiving hospitals to make critical decisions that influence a patient's treatment plan. Paramedics bring invasive procedures ordinarily done in an Emergency department of a hospital to a sick patient long before they ever arrive at the hospital.

So who are we? I used to think that there was this natural progression similar to a career ladder , starting as a firefighter and working your way to firefighter/EMT. Then once they've seen it all and have plenty of experience the EMT goes back to school and becomes a paramedic. When I was in elementary school, the fire department would visit our school in October during Fire Prevention Week and give tours of the fire apparatus. They would explain what the variety of equipment did and how different tools were used. When I'd see a fire engine screaming down the street, I had a pretty good idea what they were going to do and how they did it. Obviously I was not educated to the level of one of the firefighters on the apparatus, but I had a general concept of the work they do. An ambulance was exciting to see making its way down the street too, but I had no idea how in depth the work of the clinicians on board was. Simply put, it is such an understated service. I just didn't have the exposure to it.

I still believe there is not enough public education pertaining to the Emergency Medical Services (EMS). The public knows that when somebody is sick or injured, they should call the emergency phone number and in minutes there will be a few people at the house with a stretcher to whisk the patient off to the hospital. Beyond that, few people have the firsthand knowledge or other education to inform them of the roles and responsibilities of the providers on the inside of the flashing box truck.

When we're in public places grabbing a snack because we haven't had the ability to eat a sit-down meal, people don't know how to greet us. We have the advantage of fitting into an umbrella concept of emergency services. We hear a lot of "Thank you for your service" or "Be safe out there." I am genuinely appreciative

when somebody recognizes us for the job we have and takes just a

second to say a quick little cliché to remind us that we aren't

invisible. But occasionally, the conversations take a darker, more

morbid turn.

"What is the worst thing you have ever seen?"

I don't care if it's your first day or you're reading this after

retirement, you know what the worst call of your career was. You

flash to that scene when you encounter a certain smell. You have

the same day every year that is an anniversary you'd rather forget.

You pass that intersection, house, nursing home, bridge, landmark,

whatever the setting was; and you remember every detail of that

moment. You remember how you felt. You remember how bad

you were tested. You remember who your first phone call was to

and probably the entire transcript of that conversation.

It was a Friday morning in July. We were watching TV in

disgust as investigators were going in and out of a movie theater in

Colorado after a tragedy unfolded during the premier of *"The Dark Knight Rises."* At 1035 we were dispatched for cardiac arrest. Immediately after dispatch the county advised it was a three-year-old male in a pool found floating by a neighbor.

I got behind the wheel of the ambulance and could probably to this day still navigate myself there. The whole way there I was driving with one hand and cleaning out my pockets with the other to be ready to dive into the pool.

The fire department and paramedics beat us there and got the boy out of the water and were attempting to resuscitate him in the yard next to the swimming pool. The back door flew open and his mother rushed out toward everyone. I held her back so that she would not injure anybody and explained what was going on. We scooped him up and loaded him into the ambulance. I had no idea who all I had in the back of the ambulance, but there were more people than I started with. I just burned rubber the whole way to the hospital. We were not taking time to park so I pulled straight up to the entrance.

The trauma team met us inside and took over resuscitation.

Twenty minutes went by. I watched from the foot of the table and

made contact with his lifeless little eyes. Water was still leaking

out of his mouth as they did compressions. The attending doctor

shook her head periodically acknowledging defeat. She called out

the time of death. I left to clean up the ambulance.

Family was beginning to arrive at the hospital. Their grief

could be heard in the form of loud wailing and screaming in

disbelief clear across the campus. Nurses were walking out in

tears, seasoned healthcare providers weeping like children. When

we returned to the station, there was silence. We went about our

day completing our chores, and I honestly don't remember if we

had any more calls that day. We had nothing but time to sit and

dwell on what happened.

There was no pow wow to review the call. There was no

checking on each other. There was no interaction at all. Even our

chief and supervisor stayed in their office and conducted business

as usual. Was there no chaplain for the company to be able to sit with us and offer some comfort even if I couldn't accept prayer at

this time in my life? I felt like I had been the only one affected at

all by this.

At one point I called my girlfriend at the time to tell her

that I'd just had the worst call of my career. I told her what

happened and she replied, thanking me for ruining her day too. I

hadn't called necessarily looking for sympathy from her, rather a

listening ear to get it off my chest, but she made it abundantly clear

that she had no sympathy to offer if I had been. I was alone in my

feelings and felt like I couldn't talk to anybody.

The night before, I had been sitting in a classroom at the

local community college listening to the information session for

the paramedic program. I had been looking forward to furthering

my education and making a long career of this, but now I wasn't

sure I actually wanted to.

At the end of that Friday, we had shift change. When the

EMT for night shift came in and picked up the pager to review the calls from the day, she kept repeating how sad that run was. She'd heard about it. But she wasn't there. *She* was sad? I cussed her out and left. I was done with this. I was also beginning to consider other lines of work. I was ready to throw it all away.

You never forget calls like these. This was the first time I had seen a child die, and I did not take it well at all. I was left to stay inside my head all day until her words set me off. And yet nobody ever reached out to me about the call, my outburst, or where my head was at. Nothing was addressed.

A month later I used my VA benefits to speak with a counselor for a couple sessions. She pointed me in the direction of meditation. By that time, though, I had already pushed so many other people away and isolated myself. The bar was more attractive than my girlfriend. I didn't want to open up to anybody and show weakness, but the weakness culminated when I was stuck in a dream sleep-walking and ended up urinating on the floor next to my roommate's bed. I woke up to my other roommate cleaning up the puddle while I was standing over him.

The Double-Edged Sword

I never did receive closure. The little boy's body was cremated, and the funeral home told me years later that he had not been buried in a cemetery. I couldn't even leave him a teddy bear at his final resting place.

So no, I don't answer this inquiry from the public. I like to respond "my paycheck" and then turn and walk away. I don't understand why people don't think about the impact of a question like that. To me, it's the equivalent of asking a military veteran if he ever killed anybody. In both cases, we're not proud of those moments. My advice to anybody in EMS who has that bad call that will stick with them for the rest of their life is to come up with a quick remark as an abrupt end to a conversation that never should have started.

I have come to accept that the public maintains a curiosity about what we do. Maybe they feel that hearing an in-depth re-creation will help them comprehend what exactly it is we do. Regardless, it's not fair to put yourself in that position to have to relive something like that, especially if it was recent and you still don't understand where you're at with working through it.

The other dark side to public interactions is this perception that we are there to grab a Yoo-hoo, a Snickers, and a sandwich and hand out medical advice. There are people who will stand between us and our lunch to share about their own recent trauma, or surgery from ten years ago, or their most current change to their medications. In most cases, these are complete strangers who engage us and who we will never encounter again. I think it's so bizarre how we keep our heads down in public to accomplish whatever it is we are setting out to do without being interrupted by somebody with a question or story, but at the same time, we rush into the privacy of a stranger's home to ask the most personal questions and get very hands-on with people who have called us there in the worst moments of their day.

The fact remains that at any given time throughout our shift we can walk into somebody's crisis, operate as a team, provide high-intensity patient care, deliver this package to the hospital, and then just reset. We function on adrenaline. When somebody is having a heart attack in front of you and your hands are going a mile a minute obtaining information, administering drugs, starting IVs, and collecting labs, there is no greater satisfaction than knowing that the work you are doing at that moment is going to significantly decrease the delay between arrival at the hospital and definitive cardiac therapy. You give it everything you have, and then you turn it off. You restock, reset, and drive back to your starting point ready to do it all over again.

So day after day over the length of your career you and a partner or a small crew deliver this kind of high-quality care together. This develops camaraderie like no other. You go through these situations that nobody else will understand. You all come together and collectively experience this run and mitigate whatever is thrown at you. There is a tight unspoken bond that develops which will be there your whole life.

Chapter 2: Sowing roots

I was young, a sophomore in high school. It was late and I was getting ready for bed because I had to catch the school bus in the morning. My dad was still by the TV, probably already sleeping instead of going back to his own bed. The pager beeped loudly. The narrated address was between Dad's house and the firehouse. My fire company was being dispatched to assist with a cardiac arrest. Dad shot up out of his seat, and I was dressed and out the door in seconds. Dad knew the street and took me right to the house. We arrived at the same time as the ambulance. Joe was on the crew and had his hands full of equipment moving briskly to the front door where a woman in her 80s stood in a negligee, an image that still haunts. She held open the door as we barreled into her home and made our way upstairs to her husband lying naked on the bedroom floor. He wasn't breathing and had no pulse, so as instructed by Joe, I began chest compressions. He inserted an airway adjunct into the patient's mouth and used an Ambu bag to breathe for him. I was nervous doing CPR for the first time, but Joe talked me through it. We kept our count and rhythm in line with the defibrillator and followed the prompts given when necessary. This man and woman had just finished having sex together. She'd gone to the bathroom and heard an odd sound from the bedroom and walked back to find him dead on the floor. I promise you one thing. When I was sitting in class at the firehouse getting CPR-certified, this was not the scenario I had in mind for my first time actually needing to do CPR.

This particular call engaged my curiosity. I had a job to do, but I was also watching everyone else in their roles. More and more people were entering and doing different things with medications and breathing tubes and stuff that was way over my head. When the ambulance left for the hospital with the man in the back, I climbed into Dad's van and we drove home. I went to bed that night not knowing the outcome, not educated at all in what happened next.

A few months later, I heard that the firefighters at my company could ride along with the ambulance. We could sign up for a shift to shadow the crew and see what it was like to do their job. It worked out for me that the crew I was assigned to was with Joe. Their shift started before I got off my school bus, and I relied on my dad to take me to their station when he got home from work. By that time, they had two emergencies to handle and were in their tight little office discussing the runs together as they documented their treatments. This was a Thursday night which was memorable because the TV show *ER* still had new episodes on

NBC on Thursday nights. Joe walked out of the office and told me

to get ready. He said *ER* comes on in a half hour, and it never fails

that the local nursing home calls every Thursday night right around

the time the show starts. This was my introduction to EMS

superstition, but as warned we were out the door five minutes

before the show started to take somebody out of the nursing home

and to the hospital.

I made it a point to ride along regularly with Joe. He and

his partner Michelle always explained the hows and whys to me

really well and seemed to enjoy having me along. They will go

down in history as my biggest influences in getting into EMS.

Years later I would have the privilege of working side by side with

Joe at another service. It was a job offer I couldn't turn down.

EMS shifts range from 8 hours to 36 or more hours long.

When I began working at the transport service, I could be

partnered up with anyone and everyone on a day-to-day basis, no

rhyme or reason. Mostly luck of the draw. I had the opportunity

to get to know all of my coworkers to some extent and from there build up meaningful relationships. When I was hired on at the hospital-based service, I was assigned to a platoon with a handful of staff whose work schedules were the same, and we changed stations, shifts, and partners on some kind of set rotation among only a handful of the staff. We had closeness as a platoon, and some of my best friends came from here. When you work this closely with individuals for that long of a shift, you have to have a great working relationship so that you can bounce ideas off each other and figure out when either of you is having a bad day.

Years later, as a new dad and getting ready for my wedding, I had taken a job offer from a private sector EMS organization that offered free benefits for the whole family. At this agency, I was guided through orientation and brought up to the organization's policies by Tommy. Tommy was a seasoned medic with the organization with plenty of tenure. He not only led me in my transition but also helped me to knock on God's door for the first time.

The Double-Edged Sword

Through the local Assembly of God church, there were a few ordained chaplains who were cross-trained in CPR and who rode on the ambulance as an additional crewmember. They always seemed to find their way to the patients who needed them most, and they were always around for the providers after a challenging call.

On Sundays, Tommy and I would try to get on the same ambulance together as we would attend the morning contemporary service at the church our chaplains came from. I had not been close to a church in years. Attending that service each Sunday was one of the best choices I made in a long time. Tommy's wife would join him there. Chaplain Fred, who married my wife and me, would sit in the row ahead of us with his wife. Pastor Curtis (EMS/Police Chaplain as well) would lead the service and often had a message that was meshed together with experiences with the police and EMS chaplains. It was a welcome start to a Sunday shift because Sunday shifts were often my worst.

Anybody who comes into this job is brought up by a team of providers who will help to educate, train, and make the provider a better version of themself. Everyone we encounter has something to offer us. As you build on the educational foundation of the job, senior providers will share their tips and tricks to offer shortcuts or a more thorough way of documenting or just a different mentality to the overall approach. They've experienced things differently and have adapted to their experiences, as these things have shaped the provider they ultimately became. In much the same way, I believe that everybody we contact in our lives is put there with a purpose as well. I believe this theory applies to all aspects of our lives, regardless of the faction people assign themselves to. In the emergency services, we adapt pieces of our partners to ourselves and to the type of clinician we will ultimately become.

Chapter 3: Interpersonal Challenges

As Tommy and I were traversing a back mountain road, he was talking to his wife on the phone. We had at least fifteen minutes between the time we left our station and when we would arrive at the patient that needed us. In the back of our ambulance, Chaplain Fred was riding quietly, preparing himself to cater to the family. We arrived at the scene where a six-year-old boy with developmental problems had fallen into cardiac arrest. As an EMT it was my job to do CPR while the paramedic provided advanced cardiac life support techniques and would ultimately make the call when it was time to stop the heroic efforts. That day I was the paramedic in charge. Tommy and I got into the back of the ambulance where the little boy was laid out on the stretcher with a pair of EMTs, exhausted from their efforts, diligently working on this child. Outside the ambulance, Chaplain Fred was talking with the boy's family. Tommy was at my side to assist with meds and airway interventions as needed while supporting the overall resuscitative attempt. The cardiac monitor indicated that there was no cardiac activity despite almost an hour of resuscitation. It was time to make a decision. It was now on me to call the doctor and get the order to stop efforts on this boy. With my voice cracking, I reported everything that had been done so far and ultimately acknowledged the order by the doctor to stop.

I exited the ambulance, walked down the driveway and down the street. I knelt down in a roadside ditch and cried. This six-year-old boy's life had been cut short, and there was nothing I could do to stop it. I called my wife. I was unaware that at the time she answered the phone to my wailing she was sitting in the

car in the drive-thru lane of the bank with a suddenly very

confused teller on the other end of the microphone.

With Alaina's background in EMS, she understood where I

was coming from and was able to offer the support that I needed at

that moment. By the end of the phone call, Tommy and Fred had

found me and walked with me back to the truck having already

requested to our chief that I take the rest of the day off.

So many times I've had to accept that bad days happen.

And when they do, it's important to have a solid support structure

in your life to back you. I had that in both Fred and Tommy. I had

it with my wife. I had it in other colleagues who had experienced

struggles with me in the past. They were only a phone call away.

This was not the first time a patient had died or that I had to

terminate resuscitation. This was not the worst call of my career.

The difference with this call was that it was my first time in charge

of pronouncing a child. These are the hardest calls for EMS

providers. We see the innocence of a child and can't wrap our minds around why they deserve to die. The importance of having

someone to check on you after calls like these cannot be

overstated. So often it takes a long time for the providers involved

to recover and find peace in the situation *if* that peace *ever* comes.

Going back to the first chapter where I mentioned the

public asking 'what is the worst thing you've ever seen,' it's

important to note that we don't just hold onto the worst things. We

carry big victories with us. We carry challenging scenes with us.

We are shaped by the obstacles we've overcome. The struggles we

hold onto and the things that excite us are much different than the

average person.

I wasn't long into being a paramedic, just approaching my

first year anniversary of taking my certification tests, when my fire

company was dispatched as part of a technical rescue team to stand

by in station to possibly assist with an incident in a neighboring

county. A vehicle had been driving, and when the road turned, the

van crashed into an old mill on the side of the road. This particular

day I had agreed to go in early for my night shift so that my dayshift counterpart could attend an event. I was already in

uniform and ready to walk out the door to go to work. When the

dispatch came in, I identified the intersection to be in my zone at

work. Knowing that this had the potential to be a long night, I

drove my vehicle directly to the scene where the fire departments

were staging so that I could take over patient care and my

counterpart could get out when he needed to and drive my car back

to station.

When I walked up to meet him face to face, he told me that

this was a one-in-a-million. The mill had been built on a hill in the

1700s or earlier and was no longer operational, more a historical

landmark. The van had crashed into the upper level and collapsed

the floor, dropping headfirst into the lower level. The van itself

was a wheelchair van with a powered ramp inside the sliding side

door. The driver was in a motorized wheelchair pinned between

his wheelchair and the steering wheel. The chair would not turn on

because it detected that it was not on a level surface. The other

medic stayed outside and subsequently left as I made my way

inside the mill where the collapse team had begun their work. The driver kept telling me to let him go, afraid that the whole mill was going to collapse. I climbed in the van with him and had verbal communication with members of the collapse team who were shoring up the upper level with cellar jacks and struts.

The driver had not been injured severely in the crash, but his wrist did get stuck between the armrest of his chair and the console by the shifter. His challenges were not medical, but getting him out was going to be a slow, meticulous process of ensuring safety and being creative in extricating him from the van without further injuring him or putting him in harm's way. I called for our helicopter as protocol dictated that one acceptable use of the helicopter was for extended extrication times in a rescue. We definitely checked that box.

It's important to mention here that during my paramedic curriculum we had a rescue day. We were rappelling down the side of the drill tower and crawling through a simulated urban collapse scenario having dirt kicked on us and water dumped on us with little to no light while dragging bags with us to find and

"treat" patients (mannequins). It was late October, cold, and I had

been at a Halloween party the night before where I was up very

late and drank with a whole bunch of my friends. I had to be up

early the next morning to go through these rescue scenarios, and it

was cold. I made it very clear that I was not in the mood to do this

stuff because I would never do this type of rescue stuff. It wasn't

my intention to join the technical rescue team in the capacity of a

paramedic.

So there I was sitting in a van with a man who had

demonstrated that luck really was not on his side that particular

day. I had called for the helicopter which already had application

with the technical rescue team as many of the staff were trained to

the rescue discipline, and they would fly a cache of medications

and surgical instruments to the scene for a large-scale rescue where

resources would be exhausted.

The helicopter landed, and the first thing I wanted to know

was who was on it. Incident Command told me that my first

favorite person Liz was on. She was a flight nurse, the nicest lady

in the world. If she knew you and hadn't seen you in a while she

would always give a smile and a hug first thing when she landed

on your scene. She cared so deeply for her coworkers and all of us

she encountered regularly. Then I was told my new [just now]

favorite person was the flight medic. He was David, one of the

instructors of the rescue paramedics. I told the team I wanted him

inside with me.

When David got inside the van with me, he surveyed the

vehicle to see what was intact and what wasn't. He was looking

for anchor points to try to start making pulley systems to get the

driver out of his pinned state. During the next hour, I watched

intently and learned as David essentially assembled a crane in the

back of the van to lift the very heavy power chair off the driver.

That was only the first challenge.

We worked diligently to get the driver secured to a

backboard in this tiny space and then hoist him up through his van,

out the back window, up through the hole he created in the floor, and out to the stretcher waiting at the exterior wall where he came

crashing through. All the while, Liz was peeking through cracks in

the wood and stone construction checking on us and talking to us

to make sure we were being safe. We mitigated this together, and

it was definitely one of the most challenging and educational runs I

have ever been on. Michelangelo had the Sistine Chapel. I had the

wheelchair van in the mill.

In the off-hours when we are not working, we socialize like

everybody else. I've personally found that different social circles

aren't always the most beneficial thing. Referring back to the fact

that the general public doesn't understand what we do, we often

have gaffes in conversations that make people uncomfortable or

put off. While it's nice to hear about other things besides work, it

is an area to approach with caution.

My father-in-law used to host a Super Bowl party for his

friends and employees at his house. These were people from all

walks of life in one place. When someone asks what you do for a

living and you respond "paramedic", the reactions are all over the place. Some people think back to the television series *Emergency*

and are inquisitive about different rescue scenarios you've been in.

Some fall into that earlier category of the overbearing public.

Sometimes there's a nurse or medical assistant in the room who

has the need to one-up any of your experiences with a story about

difficult cases that walked into their controlled environment of an

office.

Our job demands that we are up to date with clinical

studies, best practices, current protocols, and situational awareness.

We educate ourselves both formally in a classroom setting with

some sort of regularity or we study online to broaden our

knowledge. We don't always have something to contribute to

conversations about investments because we don't have time to sit

and read the business journals. We can't always relate to a group

of business people or a group of manual laborers. We have our

niche.

Sometimes people will just ask about different ethical

challenges we face and how we mitigate them in an endless array of "what if" questions. The best part of being a paramedic is never

having to address the elephant in the room because we *are*

oftentimes that elephant.

In many cases, our friends outside of work are the same

people we are with at work. We bond over the runs we have been

on together. We talk about the fires we assisted on. We joke about

the stressors that we encounter, and we understand each other

without long explanations about the jargon we use, in much the

same way as members of the military remain bonded after war.

In my younger years, I had a vast number of relationships

with girls who were otherwise "normal." (Stay with me here.)

They had jobs that everyone else had with hours that everyone had

and with the same concerns everyone had. One of the challenges

in maintaining these relationships was that when they got home at

the end of their work day, leaving on time with all their colleagues,

their day was done. When they logged off their computers, the

emails were still at work waiting for the next day. The project was

stored on a drive somewhere for them to return to later. The spreadsheets, the inventories, the payroll, the veterinary records,

whatever it was, was there for the next day.

The only thing missing was that their boyfriend was still

with the volunteer fire company at somebody's burning house and

would miss the dinner plans. Five minutes before the end of shift,

just as I'm thinking about my plans after work, somebody might

collapse in their own dining room. Instead of going home, I'm

now taking care of them throughout a long, arduous clinical

encounter that is going to take a long time to mitigate and

document. The only reliable part of our schedule is that if we are

not there when our shift starts, we will be marked late. The written

end of our shift is only the report time for the next shift of workers.

You get home when the work is done. This is true of police,

firefighters, and EMS workers.

In my experience I have not been an easy person to date. I

wouldn't make plans within three hours of the end of my

scheduled shift. I compared my value as a person to the number on

my paycheck, so I always felt inadequate meeting parents for the first time. How could I support their daughter on these wages? I spent my whole day on an adrenaline rush releasing endorphins into my system all day. People relied on me, high-fived me, educated me.

The struggle I found is that for the length of my shift, I had been going from one adrenaline-filled scene to the next to the next. To get home at the end of the day to a hot meal was always nice. Going to the movies or going for a walk wasn't exactly thrilling. Nothing really was. Where was the adrenaline? What could we talk about?

I was a firm believer that you don't date coworkers because if it didn't work out, you still had to face each other at work with other coworkers put in the awkward position of having to pick sides. So how was anybody to understand my stories about my day? How could I expect anyone to understand why I didn't want to go back out once I got home? Sometimes I would skip out on the girlfriend altogether to go to the firehouse and sit and wait for an emergency to be reported to keep the adrenaline going.

It is very common for an EMT or medic to be dating or married to a firefighter or nurse or cop. These jobs share the same hectic days, odd hours, and understanding of each other's stories. In addition to the excitement of each other, they get to hear about each other's days and share stories with mutual understanding and excitement.

Coming home to tell a tale of a patient with a tracheotomy who was slowly suffocating in a nursing home would consist of details about vital signs and conditions of the site of the procedure and appliance. These tend to be very descriptive details. So if I'm sitting down to dinner with a retailer and her family, the climax of the story is going to be received very poorly when all it took to fix this patient was to suction out a mucous plug with some of the oddest shades of yellow and green that I have ever seen in my life. This story would be a total mood-spoiler to the wrong audience.

In the wrong company, a question like "How was your day?" becomes a simple "Fine." So how then do you establish a solid foundation of communication in the dating phase to take the relationship further? Sometimes it was just easier to take care of physical desires than waste time trying to establish an emotional connection since the communication is clearly doomed from the start, right? Herein lies the start of a downward cycle of behaviors that lead to issues with selfishness, ego, and ultimately fidelity.

I also decided at this point that I didn't really need to have guy friends outside of the firehouse and through work. These were people who were in a position to always have your back in very poor conditions. They were needed friendships in the heat of the moment for survival. Off the job and socially, guys were in competition. If I began to take an interest in a girl at a bar or a chance meeting, I would have a group of guys with similar interest flexing their own egos, pursuing their own desires like a pack of wolves on the hunt to establish the alpha male.

Instead, I made my pursuits on my own. I'd reach out and go out on my own towards whatever the pursuit of the week was this time. If anything began to materialize, I might bring her around the guys, but at that point there was already some kind of connection, so the competition was no longer a variable. I was all eyes on the prize without much regard for the people closest to me.

Conquest after conquest only satisfied one need. She might stay around for a while, but it was only a matter of time before she was gone. She might want more, but I couldn't accept that. After years of living on emotional pleasure at work and physical pleasure in the off time with a huge separation of the two, it seemed like I was completely addicted to pleasure. I never had to have difficult conversations about relationships. I never had to adjust my schedule for anyone. Days of the week were filled with names like appointments on a schedule.

Having not gone to college straight out of high school, I missed out on the part of life where you develop close social bonds through fraternities or other social clubs. I was hanging out at firehouses with people twice my age in some cases. The way I was supposed to act in different groups was decided by the makeup of the group. Among those of us who were younger we could be a little rowdy and have fun. The older members didn't carry the same appreciation for such behavior. In their presence you

behaved yourself accordingly. When tempers flared and clashes

occurred, I would cower away. I had no aptitude for confrontation.

It was easier to dodge responsibility and avoid any confrontation

altogether.

What I couldn't see then is that the anxiety was already

building up inside me, unnoticed. I had effectively taken myself

out of contention for any happy, meaningful future. Instead I

chased every temptation: alcohol, sex, money. I used people only

to inflate my own ego. When you hit rock bottom morally, you

find that you have sold yourself to the devil and have been driven

by only lust and pride. I am only one person who faced these types

of relationship struggles in a career a million strong. How many

other people did I know that were also struggling like me? It

wasn't about them. It was all about *me*.

Some of my best mentors in EMS were also facing demons

I never knew about. The coworkers with demons similar to mine

were the ones I would hang out with when I chose to do so.

Successful wolves hunt in packs. If I wanted to hang out with the guys, we would go to the bar, seduce suitors for the evening with our stories of great victories--pulling a person out of a burning building, bringing the dead back to life, cutting apart vehicles that were hiding injured people inside them. We took on the best version of our own realities to idolize ourselves and to pursue lustful desires. I'll never know the actual ratio of girls who bought the heroic tall tales versus girls who were just as broken as us, trying to fill a void.

It was a very slippery rabbit hole to fall down; but I believe it had to happen for me to gain perspective. The funny thing about hitting rock bottom is the false hope that you can only go up from there. There is no solace in being there. When you don't have positive support in your life, a phone call to an ignorant girlfriend about the death of a child turns into being chastised for ruining her day. And when that breakup occurred, her final life advice to me was "Don't kill any more kids." Rock bottom gets deeper.

The Double-Edged Sword

Chapter 4: Observing the Word

The siren was screaming intersection after intersection. We were only receiving information as the call-taker was entering information into the computer that was pertinent to EMS. With no communication with police, we were partially blind. We were driving quickly to get to a safe place near the address of a shooting. The dispatcher relayed that the police had declared the scene safe. We entered to find a middle-aged woman with a gunshot wound through her temple, and with a larger wound on the other side of her head. The hot lead bullet had lodged itself in the ceiling. Her daughter sat in the living room, holding onto a letter from her mother telling her how much she loved her.

When the chaplain arrived, he listened intently as the daughter reported events of the day. My partner that day, a mother of many children, was also the designated mother for our company. She was always the one who would check on you first after a bad call. She was the one you could vent to without your frustrations being spread far and wide. She stood with this girl wiping her tears and offering bottled water while she talked with the chaplain. I sat in the ambulance, ipad in hand, and did my paperwork for this run. In this moment of profound mourning, Pastor Curtis looked at the girl and offered to pray with her.

Amidst his prayer and his counsel, he looked her in the eyes and said, "If you had known that on this day, at this time this would happen, you would have moved mountains to prevent it." These words have stuck with me and remain a powerful memory from this scene. In that moment he visibly eased the guilt on that girl's face. As if she had a deep spiritual epiphany, she stopped

blaming herself. This is not to say that her mourning was over; but

from that moment, she never once repeated that it was her fault for

not being home when it happened. His words came from his heart

or maybe a spirit even deeper than that. I couldn't understand how

his words could have such a profound impact. Several months

later I had an invitation to lunch with him so we could talk through

some thoughts.

So many times I had sat in his sanctuary and heard him

speak of miracles in booth 1 of Panera Bread Company. He would

meet with people seeking hope and answers, people who turned to

the church to find healing from some horrific life traumas they

incurred. He would describe the painful events that led to their

meeting and then rejoiced in their decision, "right there in booth 1

of Panera Bread" to turn their lives over to Christ. He told these

stories so often in his messages with such conviction. Now here I

came with an invitation to that very booth.

The Double-Edged Sword

We talked about my life. We talked about my career. We discussed some of the calls we had been on together. He asked me where I stood with Christ. I told him I was a Christian, and I got saved in middle school at a youth group event. But I hid behind the shield I'd raised with all of the years of lustful pursuits hidden behind me. I thanked him for lunch and we went about our day. No miracle in booth 1 for me.

When we work this job, we don't always consider the spiritual side of things. We understand anatomy and physiology as the top contributor to how we do our job. Unless we attend a religious college or university, religion and spirituality aren't taught.

Science has led to the development of the protocols and treatment modalities used in emergency medicine. We see how molecules react and we know how the body is anatomically formed through atoms and bonds. We know that every living cell has a carbon atom, characteristic of every organic piece of matter. Our education pursues to drive home the physiology of illness as well

50

as normal body function. When something creates a shift in the overall homeostasis of the human body this is step one of the ability for a disease process to overtake. This can be caused by inside or outside stimulus. The body is a dynamic mass of tissue and cells specialized into the human described in a textbook. Our job prepares us to treat the textbook version of a human. We know why stuff happens to the body, and we have a history of traditional approaches to treating the ailments founded on anecdotal and evidence-based science. When you focus on treating illness and injuries from that perspective, this is the easiest job in the world. No transference or disappointment. When we see a problem with somebody's breathing, we look at the rate of breaths per minute, changes in heart rate, quality of the sounds in their lungs, and distal tissue changes. We gather all this evidence and fit it into a predetermined course of treatment. If there's fluid in the lungs, get it out. If the heart isn't functioning, make it pump. Blood goes round and round, air goes in and out; any deviation needs addressed.

When you follow this mentality you become a tool. You are one piece of a machine that will be used to fix a problem. As part of an assembly line, you show up, do your job, leave, sleep, wake up, return, do your job, etc. If this is the approach you follow you're set up to have an easy career. If you fix it, great. If not, there will be more opportunities.

However, we often don't function this way because we are human. We have our judgment, common sense, concern, empathy. We have our spirit who makes us the person we are. We carry our ego with us on our shoulders. When we do our job with great outcomes, we boost our ego. When we fail, we fix the problem and come back harder to get the reward of the boosted ego. We have a humanistic approach. We *are* humans.

The scientific wad of atoms in front of us is also human, so in addition to addressing all that science has proven to us, we also have to treat the person. Nobody calls an ambulance for help because they've just had the best day of their life and it's getting better. They call at their worst. They're anxious, scared, in pain, and sometimes not in their right frame of mind. Some disease processes alter the mind and mental status. Of course the best part is most people haven't read the textbook. They will report their experience, not the textbook.

We spend so much money getting educated to the science which sometimes scratches the surface of psychology, but the bottom line is if we become so consumed in *our*selves and *our* egos and *our* priorities we lose our bedside manner. This is the one single most important skill of *any* clinician. If you can't connect to the patient, how can you expect them to open up and tell you everything that is going on? They have egos too. They are people too. When we fail to make the connection, we fail to thoroughly assess the problem. We end up treating the symptoms and doing nothing for the cause.

With the added luxury of having a chaplain along to treat the spiritual needs of the patients we responded to, it was helpful to quickly make a connection as a crew and then prioritize treatments after a thorough assessment. Regardless of a patient's religious denomination or spiritual status, they found comfort in having the chaplain present.

So when we attach ourselves to lust, greed, and pride we will fail to connect in our relationships time after time after time in a vicious cycle. When we block out our support networks and try to face it alone or just do it our way, what do we learn? We *can* take the negative feedback and sort through it to pick up the pieces and try again. From the clinical example, we already decided that this is not the way to go. Ultimately we lose ourselves.

Sitting in that booth at lunch was symbolic of a hand reaching out to me saying let me help. Instead, I continued on my path, knowing that what I was doing was working for me. It was *my* plan. If it wasn't broken, why fix it?

Chapter 5: The Older I Got, The More People I Thought I Knew

.

I saw a paramedic from my childhood who my parents greatly respected. He was a proud and confident man. He was funny and always had an off-colored joke ready to go. John was known throughout the community by name, even if only by reputation. As an EMT, I would walk into somebody's house where somebody was very sick and the family would ask if *he* was coming too. In one case I remember a story about a woman who was in labor who was asking for him by name. Some people knew of him by his innuendo-based nickname "Dr. Feelgood." So when a pregnant woman was asking for *him* the EMT's knee-jerk reaction was to ask if he is the father.

I had no family relation to John. I just had been brought up knowing that he was somebody you wanted to grow up to be. Everyone loved him at the pool parties I used to attend with my parents. He was a firefighter with his own local fire company but welcome at any fire scene in a 40-mile radius to help out. He was a loving father to his son, who admired him so greatly. He did his job his way and had local fame for it. I have a photo of him taking a selfie with one of our TV news reporters. I put John up on a pedestal. He was not one to accept new paramedics to train with him because he was very particular in the way he did his job and had little patience for some *new* guy trying to tell him how it was supposed to be done according to the book they just graduated from.

Christopher Turnbull

When I was doing my field training, John and I had a day together. He told me stories about my dad in the fire service, and he was very strict in how he wanted each detail of the job executed. He had very specific expectations for documentation so that a patient care report didn't get you in a courtroom defending a vague outline of the patient encounter. John was a god among men. I always thought of him this way. I had been idolizing this man for as long as I could remember for his aggressive approach to patient care and for the stern arrogance he brought to the patient care environment. As an EMT I had fear instilled in me by this man because I always felt that no matter how good I tried to be it would never be good enough for him when he arrived on scene. He would very openly tell you what you had done wrong. When you're the best of the best, you don't need to be polite.

One fact that cannot be overstated is how much love John had for his son, an EMT taking classes to become a paramedic. When they would cross paths in the hospital ER he would always wrap his arm around his son's shoulders and kiss him on top of his

57

head and tell him he loved him. It never seemed to matter what else he was up to at the moment. One time I was working with his son who was in the bathroom first thing at the start of shift. John stopped by our station as he was driving back to his station. He came inside looking for his son, so I directed him. He knocked on the door and told him he loved him and left to go about his day. What a guy!

Years later, I would learn that John was involved in some kind of altercation with his fifth wife (I don't think I ever realized he was married) which ended abruptly as he shot her in the driveway before going out the back of his house and shooting himself.

When this happened, I heard of it over the phone from one of our former coworkers. I was in the parking lot of Wal-mart in Ocean City, Maryland, driving in lazy circles as my son and daughter napped in their car seats in the back of the car. My wife was inside gathering a few items we needed. I'll never forget that moment. The man who I wanted to grow up to be like in so many ways had a whole personal life that I knew nothing about. I spent my whole life idolizing the real-life hero my father and so many others painted him to be; but I never really knew *him*. Here was somebody who I had so much contact with throughout my life, and who had been fighting so many demons in his own life. Could a single conversation have changed his path? Could I have tried harder to spend time with him off shift?

But then I wondered. At that time in my life, could I have noticed anybody struggling? Honestly, the answer is no. I was a brand-new paramedic. The ego that I carried with me up to that point was already controlling every action, thought, and plan for after work.

This is just one story of a coworker lost to suicide. Unfortunately I have more, not just coworkers. One of the mechanics who worked on our ambulances took his own life. Another paramedic from the same agency suffered through anxiety and would have debilitating panic attacks. He took his own life.

When I started my schooling to become a medic, I worked for a very small municipal ambulance company part time, which allowed me to make some money while I used the vast downtime to do my schoolwork. This was the company where I responded to the call with the little boy in the pool. Another part-time EMT there took his own life. How bad were these people suffering that it got this far?

One service that is often offered after a single stressful event is a critical incident stress management (CISM) debriefing. These are usually available following some kind of profound incident guaranteed to make the front page in the next day's newspaper. The problem is that for every once-in-a-decade incident like this for a single person, that individual has tens of thousands of unique stressors. So what are we doing for the men and women out there expected to save lives when they themselves are the ones who need help?

I think overall we do a terrible job of checking up on each other. Even with a debriefing immediately after the event, what kind of follow-up is there a week down the road? A month down the road? Why are we expected to process the whole ordeal in one open forum?

People have said to me before that they don't know how I do this job. I have never had any kind of profound answer to give. Oftentimes I've said that coffee helps. Among the right audience I've made some quirky, dark remarks. Answers like these do give some sort of acceptable explanation. People respond to stress differently. My method has led to me developing a very dark sense of humor.

How do you approach such a serious job with humor? The first thing to understand is that not every dispatched emergency is actually a life-threatening emergency. There are many anecdotes that I've heard that have come from these types of calls. Many of these calls are the source of some of my own comical stories. Among our colleagues, some of the best conversations are spent laughing at some of the most off-the-wall stories that no reasonable person could ever make up. It has been said before that laughter is the best medicine, and honestly it helps to be able to laugh through the stress.

So how do we miss the ones who are suffering? If we hold the stress inside and ignore it or overshadow it with humor, it doesn't go away. We just keep making deposits into the suppression bank and let it collect interest over time. It sits there and festers, whether we recognize it in ourselves or not. Remember our shifts are only so long. Afterwards we go home and have to live a normal life. We can't just let our feelings out. Who will understand? I can't tell my kids about my fears or my close calls. I don't want them to worry or be frightened by me going to work. We use humor to protect ourselves then suppress everything inside to protect the ones we love from the stressors we face.

My closest friends are hours away. Throughout my career, we met on the job, life changes occurred to separate us, and time is not plentiful enough to get together. Some of my friends haven't heard from me in over a year. With others, we go long periods of time between talking or seeing each other but always seem to pick up right where we left off. The important thing is we know how to reach each other when we need to.

My best friend knows to call me regardless of the time of day. I've sat on the phone with her and let her cry things out for long periods of time. She has gone through a lot in her work and personal life, and it has been my privilege to be her support when she needs me. I don't always have answers for her, but I'm always willing to listen. She tells me all the time that she should have been the best man at my wedding, and it is so unbelievably true.

The most important advice that I can give to anybody who reads this is to establish *your* support network. You *need* to have people in your life that you *can* lean on during a tough time. Immediate coworkers are by your side all the time and office gossip still happens in the emergency services; we're not immune to it. So often I've heard that a listening ear is a running mouth. If

63

you have the luxury of having a coworker you can confide in, do it.

If not, look at who you *do* have.

In EMS we have a strong hero complex. We are always fine until we aren't. We are great caretakers but poor patients. We don't talk about our feelings but expect our patients to accurately describe the sensation of the pain they are feeling in their chest. Most of us grew up with a heavy taboo about mental health that our industry is not exempt from. In most cases, something profound has to happen to show us *and* everybody around us that a problem exists. By that time the administration is involved in escorting you to get help. It should *never* get this far. If your support network is weak or you can't talk openly to the people you are closest to, it is absolutely fine to seek counseling. It is so important that I will state it again. It is absolutely fine to seek counseling. Post-Traumatic Stress Disorder and Acute Stress Disorder are just two conditions that, if left undiagnosed or untreated, can be a step down a long, lonely pathway that could lead to people making a permanent decision to end temporary suffering. You matter so much to more people than you will ever

know. If you want to change somebody's life, carry the crisis

intervention hotline phone number on you. Somebody needs it.

Perhaps you?

Chapter 6: A Family of My Own

I sat on my bunk at the firehouse staring at a newsfeed of

social media posts. I kept scrolling because I had nothing better to

do. I didn't want to do anything. Another firefighter, Matthew,

came in and told me that he was going to a Halloween party and I

was coming with him. I didn't want to. It was November 1st, a

little late to be having a Halloween party, but that wasn't why I

didn't want to go. My pickup truck was loaded up with plywood for a training class our fire company was doing the next morning, so I wasn't going to drive anywhere.

"There's a girl there who wants to meet you."

"No. Definitely not going."

It had been four months since the girl I was seeing told me not to kill any more kids. Since that time I was talking to/seeing a few different girls, and I just didn't care to be introduced to somebody who wanted to meet me. I already had my hands full.

"Come on. It's free beer."

"No."

"You can wear your Batman costume."

"Fine."

The first thing to note about this party was that all the snacks were homemade. This was a smaller house, but between the backyard, kitchen, dining room, and living room, the place was packed. I didn't recognize anybody there, so I stood in the dining room indulging in a homemade cheeseball and dipping graham

crackers into a strawberry cheesecake dip. Of course I found the

beer too.

Matthew bailed on me as soon as we got there to find this

mystery girl. Imagine Dragons radio station was playing on the

Pandora app on the TV setting a fun mood for the costumed

partygoers. By the time I saw Matthew again I had migrated to the

back porch for another beer. He walked up to me, escorting

probably the most beautiful peacock I had ever seen. He

introduced us; she and I exchanged hellos then off she ran. She

was the hostess of the party and was tending to everybody. I spent

the evening there until we left for the local bar for some karaoke.

This peacock and I finally had a couple of minutes to talk. She had

been observing me throughout the night. Apparently, I had made

some sort of impression as it was at the end of her party that I

received a kiss on the cheek. I told her to try again. She did.

I woke up at her house the next morning (If I drink, I stay).

Matthew had already left; his Halloween costume was tossed in a corner of the living room. I was late to meet at the firehouse for the training event, so I ran the four blocks to the firehouse dressed as Batman only to find they had all left without me.

If I would have pursued that girl that night, I would have hurt her so badly. I withdrew instead. I continued my course of destruction. I did help her at her place of employment over the Thanksgiving holiday weekend, but I still kept some distance. Around this same time I had graduated from the paramedic program and had begun another stressful period of orienting to the new position with my own employer. She called me up a few months later and asked me to come over. That night, she told me how she felt. She told me if I was going to see her it would have to be *only* her. I had been living a very sinful life, and I was tired of living that way. I pulled out my phone and said goodbye to every other girl I was juggling at that moment. Alaina and I were married two years and one month after the night we met.

Her words that night were the first step in climbing out of the hole that I had dug so deep for myself. From that night forward I was laser focused on her. There were no more long nights at the bar competing for conquests. She shook those demons off me. She took the piece of work that showed up at her party and made a man out of me.

Her family comes from a Catholic background. Her father is very devoted to his faith. He spends time every day with scripture. He built a very successful business and has provided well for his family. I turned to him on several occasions for advice. He himself spent some time with demons of his own. He approached me one day about a weekly seminar a local Catholic Church was hosting. He said he wanted to check it out but didn't want to go by himself. The seminar was about leading your family with Catholic principles; essentially striving to become more like Jesus. I attended with him biweekly on account of my work schedule for about 3 weeks before I stopped going. The statistics they were incorporating hit too close to home. I thought I was better than them and did not need the Catholic Church to tell me how to run my family. I didn't need help; I had my own plan.

Alaina and I were married in December by the same

Chaplain Fred that had given us both so much support during our

time at that ambulance company. A few months later, I received a

Valentine's Day card with the words "Love, the three of us." Our

daughter was fifteen months old at this point. The reality was that

at the end of that year, we would have two kids under two years

old. If that wasn't stressful enough, my wife's pregnancy was a

long, nightmarish nine months of vomiting while connected to IV

fluids and round the clock administration of anti-nausea

medications. The first med wasn't helping to stop the nausea. The

second one produced a near-psychotic side effect that put my wife

in a state of panic and a heavy feeling of impending doom. The

final one worked, thankfully, but her vomiting wasn't her only

struggle.

This was her second pregnancy. Her first one produced a

great deal of struggle as well, but she wasn't on round the clock

therapy with visiting nurses. I was scared. So often she would get

very angry with me and tell me that I didn't care about this child, that I wasn't excited for this one. One night she made an Italian dinner and did her own pasta sauce from scratch. I failed to comment on the sauce. The next day while I was at work, she called me to scold me for not noticing her effort. Some weeks later she would call me again to tell me that she had fallen down a few steps. She swore that she was okay. In my effort to understand, she informed me that she had in fact fallen from the top of the stairs to the bottom. She dislodged the baby gate at the bottom. I left work in a panic and took her to the hospital. She was bumped and bruised, but the baby was fine.

I carried the fear of losing my son for months on top of everything happening with her. I was scared every day. I still went to work and showed up for my patients, doing the best for them emergency after emergency. When I got home, I couldn't tell her about my stressful days. I couldn't tell her about my fears. My role was to do the best I could to provide for Piper and her because she was unable to work and being harassed by her supervisor who was inquiring when she was coming back to work.

My wife is the strongest person I know. Everything that has been dealt to her in life only made her stronger. I could not be more proud of her. I also could not stress her out any more than she already was.

A month before Reid was born, Alaina presented to the hospital with dizziness and a fever. She was admitted to the antepartum unit, an area in the hospital for mothers on hospital-based bed rest. They were encouraged to socialize and bake together, but they were not allowed to exert themselves, so a nurse was present to facilitate the activities and assist with physical tasks. She was also there to monitor the ladies and to pass meds while keeping the doctors updated. There was only one problem. Alaina was being tossed between doctors.

For the second time during that pregnancy, Alaina's IV site, a PICC line, was infected and she was septic. She had developed blood clots in her arm and armpit. Labor and delivery doctors would not take responsibility for her because she should have been under the care of the infectious disease specialists. The infectious disease doctors didn't want to take her on because she was pregnant on hospital-based bed rest. Her own obstetrician was trying to get her discharged, not knowing the full extent of the back and forth she was going through.

I still had to work. I still had to make life and death decisions and perform at my peak performance for every patient. I became very numb and very cold to people. The only thing I cared about was my family. I visited Alaina in the hospital every chance I had. Our chaplains from work would join us periodically. The hospital held a meeting with a whole team of doctors from labor and delivery, her obstetrician, and the infectious disease team. They began having daily meetings to coordinate Alaina's care. They started her on Vancomycin, a strong antibiotic. That night Alaina's neighbor in the unit had a medical emergency. The nurse assigned to the unit was tied up with her on the phone with the doctor and was summoning help as this patient was in a bad way.

Alaina looked at me with a very scared expression that I will never forget. She told me she felt hot all over, but her words were very slurred. Her skin became red and blotchy. Her heart rate climbed. She started with preterm contractions. I switched into paramedic mode and assessed the situation. I disconnected the medication. I was reporting to the nurse across the hallway who was already overwhelmed. I sat with Alaina to try to help keep her calm while maintaining my own cool so as not to scare her more. Inside I was screaming. I held her hand in a way that allowed me to still feel her pulse at her wrist. Alaina was becoming more and more restless. Her pulse rate was getting faster. Then it stopped.

I cycled the blood pressure on her monitor and found her pressure to be in the seventies. I updated the nurse and put my wife's bed flat with her feet elevated. Her blood pressure recovered into the nineties. The doctors came in and treated her allergic reaction. They gave her more IV fluids to bring her blood pressure back up. They assured me she was fine. I never saw the nurse that night. If I hadn't been there visiting would my wife still be alive? I was in control, remember? I was leading my family according to my plan.

The Double-Edged Sword

Reid was born healthy in October. He's currently a typical four-year-old going on fourteen. What I saw in that room that night scared me beyond anything I had ever known, and I'm a healthcare professional.

<u>Chapter 7: Life happens</u>

"One night I dreamed a dream. As I was walking along the beach with my Lord, across the dark sky flashed scenes from my life. For each scene, I noticed two sets of footprints in the sand, one belonging to me and one to my Lord. After the last scene of my life flashed before me, I looked back at the footprints in the sand. I noticed that at many times along the path of my life, especially at the very lowest and saddest times, there was only one set of footprints. This really troubled me, so I asked the Lord about it.

The Double-Edged Sword

'Lord, You said once I decided to follow You, You'd walk with me all the way. But I noticed that during the saddest and most troublesome times of my life, there was only one set of footprints. I don't understand why, when I needed You the most, You would leave me.' He whispered, 'My precious child, I love you and will never leave you. Never, ever, during your trials and testings. When you saw only one set of footprints, it was then that I carried you." --"Footprints In The Sand," Author disputed.

My in-laws were part owners of a family beach house in Ocean City, Maryland. My wife and I found ourselves traveling down every opportunity we had. Each time we visited, it was harder to leave, but we had our priorities. We had our jobs. We had our friends. I was still a volunteer firefighter and associated with the local fire company. We both had family at home, and of course we had our local spots to eat.

One morning during some waking pillow talk, Alaina asked

me if I would ever consider moving to the beach. Her parents had

bought a place not far from the family beach house to retire to.

Alaina and her mother have a very close bond. When this

conversation came up, I thought about how most people can only

dream of picking up and moving to the beach. If we were going to

consider doing this, a lot had to happen. I laid out my plan to

Alaina. We would both take a trip down to the beach house and

drive around submitting resumes. Before we could pick up and

move, we needed to have jobs. Alaina found a management

position and applied. I had found several opportunities within the

emergency services from dispatcher to firefighter to paramedic and

applied for them. Alaina took a phone interview for her position

and was later offered the job. Her start date was in the first week

of August of that year. We had two weeks to pack up our life and

make the move. We had a two-year-old, an eight-month-old, and

ourselves to pack.

The Double-Edged Sword

At the same time my dad was living his best life coming over at least weekly to play with his grandkids, have dinner served to him, and occasionally catch a campfire in the backyard. When we told him that we had decided to make this move, he was devastated.

I was fifteen when I moved in with my dad. He and I had a really good relationship. He was usually willing to get me to the firehouse quickly when an emergency was dispatched. We had season passes to a nearby amusement park and would often visit after he got home from work. My mother hated that he had custody of me and did everything in her power to chastise him as a father every opportunity she had. My dad did the very best he could to provide for me through high school. I didn't always have everything I wanted, but he was great at making sure I had everything I needed. He himself had his own share of stressors and was fighting his own demons. When my dad had a bad day at work, at least he had me to come home to. My dad had made it very clear to me that I was his rock when I lived with him.

He signed my papers during my senior year of high school, allowing me to enlist in the Army. The day I left for basic training, family was invited to see me sworn in before being bussed to the airport. My dad spent most of that day outside by himself crying. I think he aged ten years the day I took my enlistment oath and left.

When I came back and went to work full time, I wasn't around as much. He became an EMT to work with me at various events. It was the only time we really spent together. I had already discovered the path that I was headed down without realizing the destination, but as far as I was concerned I was living my best life and didn't have time for him anymore. Our interactions and time together had become awkward. We were like two strangers who had known each other our whole lives.

When I was with Alaina, that changed. She wanted to get to know him. Then when the babies came, he was always around. I got my relationship back with my dad. He had so much to look forward to. But now we were leaving.

The Double-Edged Sword

My dad still came around just as much during that window of time before our move, but we all felt the elephant in the room. It didn't take away from the attention that our kids absorbed from him, but he also didn't want to talk about it. All he asked was that we didn't ask him to help move us because he can't handle that.

When moving day arrived, we recruited some of our neighbors to help load the moving truck and the tow-behind trailer. Alaina's best friend, our matron of honor, had the kids. Walking up the sidewalk later that morning was my dad. He showed up to help us despite telling us not to ask him. That afternoon, we took back our kids. Dad spent some time with them in the car as Alaina and I finished a few last minute details. He got in his car, not without tears, and followed us onto the highway. We reached the exit that led to Dad's house, but our journey was just beginning. He passed us on the right to wave goodbye and exited the highway as we continued on with our move.

Moving is stressful. I always thought that the hard part was organizing your whole life into boxes and remembering which boxes go where. Thankfully my wife bought labels to indicate which room each box belonged in. The hard part is not packing up. The hard part is unpacking. We took every bit of two weeks to pack. Several months after the move, there were still unopened boxes in the garage, and others in the bedrooms and throughout the house we were renting. Part of the problem was that I was never around.

Alaina started her job the day after we moved in. I had some interviews, but no offers yet. My work schedule had been a two-week rotation working Monday and Tuesday during the day; off Wednesday and Thursday; working Friday, Saturday, and Sunday; off Monday and Tuesday; working Wednesday and Thursday; then off the 3-day weekend. I would leave Sunday evening from home to drive back to where we moved from and sleep in the bunk room of the ambulance company. I'd work Monday, sleep there Monday night, work Tuesday then leave to get back home very late at night. During this time, Alaina was keeping to her own work schedule with a babysitter helping out. I was away more than I was home. I continued this cycle for seven months before I got a job offer.

The year we moved, I found myself victim to a long line of bad luck. It began in February of that year. Every Sunday that I worked, I had a patient who was dead on arrival. If I took a Sunday off, I would get it the next time I worked. We were assigned to our lineup of four or five ambulances not by the truck itself but by the garage bay the truck sat in. Mine was the second from the left as you gazed outward. The farthest bay left was the start of the rotation, and that was only ever occupied when we had five ambulances in service. There are 52 weeks in a year; we worked 26 Sundays.

By late spring I was on a first name basis with the coroner himself and the majority of his deputies. My supervisor noticed that this was occurring and even changed up the rotation so that I would not be getting the first run of the morning. It didn't matter. The fact remained that if somebody was going to die on Sunday, I was going to be the one to show up.

Sunday after Sunday, I would stay in somebody's home waiting for the coroner or funeral home to arrive while family members were showing up from all over to grieve their loss as a family with their loved one still present. I heard stories of 50 years of marriage coming to an end. I heard the life story of so many of these people. On one occasion I was dispatched to a morgue to pronounce a nursing home patient dead after the overnight nurse supervisor failed to do the proper paperwork. Every Sunday I worked, somebody died.

By June I was over it. I dreaded going to work knowing that I *might* get breakfast, I *might* get the ambulance washed, but I *would* be telling somebody's spouse that their marriage is over. In some cases these were people who died in their sleep and were found the next morning when they didn't show up to church. In other cases there was a crash or other traumatic cause.

June 18th, one week before Father's Day, I had a very uneventful Sunday. I had made it through the day without being called to inform a family of their loved one's passing. I had three hours to go when I was dispatched for cardiac arrest. My partner

and I were headed for ice cream at the time, only a half-mile away

from the dispatched address. We responded to the call. Tommy,

the paramedic who trained me with the company, got in his

ambulance with his partner and also responded as it was best

practice to have a second crew along on a cardiac arrest due to the

workload associated with those events.

My partner and I arrived at the house and located a police

officer in the side yard speaking to a woman who was sitting on

the grass crying. He directed us up the steps onto the deck where

another police officer was compressing the patient's chest. The

fire department had arrived on scene and was also assisting with

CPR.

We worked on this guy for about ten minutes where we

were before we got pulses back. He remained unresponsive, but

his heart was beating on its own. Tommy was at the man's head

with a breathing tube inserted in his airway, still doing the work of

breathing for him.

I called his wife to his side and I looked her in the eyes to tell her that we had been successful in getting his pulse back. I told her that I believed he might still be able to hear her even if he couldn't respond. I told her she had a few seconds before we would be able to move him, so she had this time to talk to him.

We moved him to the ambulance and transported him to the hospital. My partner had taken over breathing for him. Tommy's partner was driving our ambulance. Tommy was following us to the hospital.

I looked up in time to see a geyser of vomit shoot up and out of the man's mouth, covering my partner's uniform. I looked back at the monitor and saw that his heart had stopped again at that moment. I turned on the Lucas device (an automated device that does uniform chest compressions making transport safer without having people standing up while the ambulance is flying down the road). I had one more syringe of Epinephrine ready to go and pushed it through the IO line that had been drilled into his leg. Not a minute later, we had pulses back again, CPR stopped, and we

arrived at the ER.

Early EKG interpretation indicated that the patient had a

heart attack. The hospital had been made aware of this and had a

team standing by to take him to the cardiac catheterization lab to

open a blocked artery to his heart. When we got into the room, the

doctor opened his eyelids and cancelled the heart cath. His pupils

were fixed and dilated. They said he was most likely brain dead

from a lack of oxygen. Fixing his heart wouldn't fix that.

His wife was brought into the room to discuss end of life

options. I was ashamed to face her. I leaned down to the patient's

ear and told him to fix himself because he worked me entirely too

hard to give up now. With that, I left the room to find my partner

and our equipment.

This was the first Sunday since February that I had been

dispatched for cardiac arrest and didn't have to tell the spouse that

their life together was over. For the next several shifts that I worked I had people check up on him for me, and at one point I

went up to his room. I found his wife standing in there over him.

She immediately recognized me and invited me in. There had been

no new update from the time that I'd left him in the ER. I felt so

obligated to say something profound to offer comfort, but I didn't

have the words. Instead I spent a few minutes with them silently

and then told her I would continue to ask about him.

Soon after, I went to Tennessee for my brother-in-law's

wedding. While I was in Nashville physically, I couldn't help

replaying the events over and over in my head. I reached out to

some of the nurses I knew to try to get updates, but ultimately I

was only creating space between me and the rest of the family and

getting no new answers. I was in no way emotionally available to

anybody there.

The day after the wedding we were to fly home. While

walking through the terminal in Nashville, my phone rang. It was

Tommy. I answered probably with my usual banter about him

being old or ugly, but he told me to hold on because somebody
wanted to talk to me.

"I don't really know what to say." The male voice on the
other end was hoarse, soft, and unfamiliar. "Thank you for saving
my life. Have a safe flight, and I'll see you soon." I was ugly-
crying in public right through the terminal, completely oblivious to
the fact that I had left my wife to push the stroller with two kids
and drag our carry-on.

As I stated before, I was done with the trend that I had set
for myself. I was tired of seeing the profound grief and mourning.
I was tired of feeling like the angel of death. I was in a dark place
and trying to decide if the work I was doing was worth it. I'd
gotten into this job to help people, but I didn't feel like I had
impacted anybody. I walked into work knowing that somebody
was going to die because it was my day to work.

"Thank you for saving my life."

Is that what happened? Or was he the one who restored my faith in myself? The reality is that I was in such a low place in my life and needed something to pick me up and lift my spirits. His amazing turnaround was exactly what I needed. So, I think it is safe to say that *he* is the one who in fact saved *my* life and career.

I had the opportunity to meet the man in the hospital when I got back. I was so impressed that he had no deficits. According to his wife, he was very much himself, off-colored jokes and all. He did eventually make it into the heart cath lab, but the findings were indicative of normal circulation. They never did find a definitive reason as to why he went into cardiac arrest that day. I heard shortly thereafter he was supposed to go to a rehab facility but instead signed out against medical advice to go home. The next time I saw him they came to our station eager to meet the four of us who had not given up on him. He had been eager to learn which one of us had been the one to whisper in his ear in the ER. He also apologized to my partner for vomiting on her. Every time I go back to visit friends, they are at the top of the list.

The Double-Edged Sword

Death is very much a part of life, and it is expected to be encountered in our line of work. At the end of the year, I had been doing my four-hour commute for four months. I had spent the last four months away from my family considerably more than I was with them. When I was home my wife wasn't most of the time because she had a work schedule too. The first two months we would go to the beach every opportunity we had, but it was cold now. There wasn't much to do.

I left late one night to go to work because I had a pounding headache. Alaina took my blood pressure, and it was very high, completely unusual for me. I was tired. I was tired of the current arrangement. I was tired of Sundays. I was tired of the anxiety.

We were taxed financially between rent, fuel, and eating out when I was at work. The stress had gotten to me. It was a tough year with moving, commuting, and Reid not sleeping through the night. I weighed 270 pounds at 32 years old. I had let myself go. Everything that I had suppressed over the last two years including Alaina's pregnancy with Reid had been weighing me down in the truest sense of the word; that and my terrible

eating habits.

I asked my supervisor to run a survey of my paperwork to

tell me how many times I had called the coroner in that year.

Again, there are 52 weeks in a year. We were scheduled for 26

Sundays. If I was off on Sunday, it caught up to me on my next

shift without fail. I had called the coroner 27 times. There wasn't

another provider that year within 15 of me. Twenty-seven times.

My father-in-law visited me on one of my days home. He

and my mother-in-law were visiting and working on their

retirement home. It was during the NFL playoffs. It was unusual

for him to be away from his TV when there was a football game

on, much less to visit me without Alaina around. He asked me if I

ever struggled with depression. He told me Alaina was concerned.

He told me he didn't know how I functioned at the pace I was

going. Of course I told him I was fine; I was doing the best I

could. I'm sure he quoted scripture to me but I can't remember exactly. He assured me I could reach out to him anytime. He told

me he loved me. Then he left.

At the end of February, I received a phone call. I finally

had a job offer and would start in the middle of March. This was

the phone call that I had been waiting on for four months. Could it

actually be true that my suffering was over?

<u>Chapter 8: Looking Up</u>

A champion named Goliath, who was from Gath, came out of the Philistine camp. His height was six cubits and a span. He had a bronze helmet on his head and wore a coat of scale armor of bronze weighing five thousand shekels; on his legs he wore bronze greaves, and a bronze javelin was slung on his back. His spear shaft was like a weaver's rod, and its iron point weighed six hundred shekels. His shield bearer went ahead of him. David asked the men standing near him, "What will be done for the man who kills this Philistine and removes this disgrace from Israel?

Who is this [giant] that he should defy the armies of the living

God?" What David said was overheard and reported to Saul, and

Saul sent for him. David said to Saul, "Let no one lose heart on

account of this Philistine; your servant will go and fight him." Saul

replied, "You are not able to go out against this Philistine and fight

him; you are only a young man, and he has been a warrior from his

youth." --1 Samuel 17: 4-7, 26, 31-33

As of my last day with the company in February, I had

functioned in the emergency services for 16 years, including my

time spent as a junior firefighter. I was well known among my

colleagues. The day I left, there were tears.

It was a bittersweet moment for me. On one hand I was

moving on and leaving all of this behind me. On the other, it was

made very clear that my time spent working did in fact impact the people around me. Not everybody, of course, but not everybody shares your perspective and celebrates your achievements.

I left with a sense of achievement knowing that I had gained the respect of so many people across our county. I looked back on some of my highlights as I drove home that day remembering the photo behind the state capitol when our region achieved teaching 250,000 people to do CPR. I recalled having the ability to move easily between agencies because I had good rapport with people from various companies. Job interviews had been a simple formality for me because administrators at least knew of me from popping up here and there over the last decade.

I had a heightened sense of pride in my accomplishments and gratuity towards the people who helped to shape me. When I began my field training to get my license issued by the new state, it was very evident that I had been a big fish in a small pond, but now I was drowning in the ocean.

The Double-Edged Sword

I came into this position carrying with me a figurative chip that had been fried in the grease of fifteen years of EMS experience. I placed that chip firmly on my shoulder for all to see. Unfortunately for me, I came in on fire, ready to take off and show everyone what I could do.

Instead, I demonstrated my proficiency at skills better than I demonstrated my overall ability to mitigate challenging patients. My evaluations were terrible. I would rush in slower than the standard ready to treat everybody. The problem was that I now had to explain every thought going through my mind. What do I see? What's going on? What's my plan? How do I execute my plan? What else can I do?

I came from a system where there was a single paramedic either driving themselves in an SUV to intercept an EMT ambulance or there was a single paramedic partnered with an EMT on an ambulance together. I was now in a system where two paramedics were partnered up to intercept an EMT ambulance. I wanted to do it all and could not change my ways to delegate tasks to my partner to expedite the patient care process.

It was a huge giant that I was facing. While I did have conditional employment for the position, I needed to demonstrate proficiency overall to the standards of the new organization. I let my pride, my ego, and my overconfidence tackle me day after day.

Eventually I began to improve on my weaknesses, little by little. Occasionally I would hit some snags on runs that proved to be setbacks. I overcame it. Seven months after my orientation phase ended and my field training phase began, I stood in front of the chief to receive my badge and my state paramedic license. For seven months, I'd pushed and pushed, facing defeat every day and not knowing if I would secure my job.

After seven months of commuting between my old job and new home, financial stress had built up beyond belief. We had not counted on that fuel expense for that length of time. That and vehicle wear and tear with the new job added up and weighed us down. I had to work overtime to catch up.

Working overtime at the new pay rate was helpful to some extent, but the childcare costs increased relatively. The first full calendar year that I had been licensed and working, I nearly doubled the salary that had been offered to me. I had become a machine. I worked at any of the stations scattered around the county as they were available or assigned to me.

The scheduled rotation was two day shifts, then two night shifts, then four days off. I was not taking four days off. We were not permitted to work a full 24-hour day due to some safety concerns that had been raised years ago, but we could work a full shift and add on half of a shift. In my thirst for money, I was scheduling myself 17 to 19 hours at a time and taking only the minimum amount of time off.

Our county is a very busy one. Depending on the station I work out of, it is possible to have 20 or more emergency calls dispatched in a 14-hour shift. I work among some of the most motivated paramedics I have ever seen. Regardless of how busy it gets, we manage our patients, restock, reset, and run out the door to the next one. We work at a grueling pace. In my short time here, I have treated some of the sickest patients I've ever encountered. The greatest part though is that I've gained so much more experience in a short three years than I feel I had gotten in four years as a paramedic previously.

The paramedic experience is different everywhere you go. Pick a place in the United States, and visit the medics. Is their area served by the shipping industry with hazards at the port? Are they in an urban setting with violent crime? Are they a rural system with long distances to drive to get to the sickest of the sick patients? Or do they have agricultural hazards? Maybe they are a small, quiet town where nothing happens. The setting of the service is a huge factor in the quality of the paramedic. Every area has its challenges, run volume, high points, and bad points. Remember, we are shaped by experience.

The Double-Edged Sword

The pace that I was working at was only ever interrupted when our friends from back home would come and visit us for a weekend. During our first summer at the beach, our house was occupied by friends every weekend. We would spend the days on the sand and in the ocean riding the waves. We'd build sandcastles with the kids and dig huge holes in the sand, playing with sand crabs along the way.

In the evenings, we would indulge in the finest dining and sometimes visit the boardwalk rides and games for some entertainment. This was the year that we realized most people save up some quantity of money to go on a beach vacation. We were trying to keep up every weekend living paycheck to paycheck. We would join our friends for that time together week after week. The excess money we were making to get caught up in life was now being diverted to a new kind of pleasure. It became an intoxicating drug for me.

During the week, we would work our jobs. I would get home at three in the morning some nights to catch some sleep and return to work again. But on the weekends when we had people

down, there was so much excitement.

On Friday, they'd be calling and texting to tell us how far

away they were. On the arrival, there were hugs and so much

anticipation for the weekend ahead. If our friends brought kids

with them, our kids shared the same excitement (if not more)

because they could finally see other kids and have a weekend-long

play date. By Saturday night we would be so deep in fun and our

hearts so warm with the fellowship we got to enjoy, but on Sunday

it was done. We'd have breakfast together, they'd pack, and by the

afternoon they were gone.

The weekend binge of activities was over, and my next

shift was hours away. This must have been what it felt like to

binge drink for a weekend then run out of alcohol. My mood was

ruined. I was literally experiencing withdrawal from fun. I began

to accept that my source of joy was outside of my home. I was so

absorbed by the money and the pleasure of spending it with our friends that I was beginning to slip away again. I found another slippery rabbit hole and dove in head first.

Alaina had wanted to go on a cruise to celebrate her 30th birthday. We booked the cruise in the summer and invited a bunch of friends to come along. Despite challenges that our latest attempt at budgeting revealed, we paid it off to embark in March. The second week of March came. We were packed and ready to go. We had loaded up the car and the kids and were heading off to our friends' house to drop off the kids until my mother-in-law could pick them up and take them for the week.

We had been listening to current events for weeks following the story of a virus. The closer we got to departure day, the more of Alaina's friends that had backed out of the trip. We were still going though. We needed this time in the Caribbean together to relax. We had special dinner plans arranged for the night of Alaina's birthday. We had all these plans.

I had been working really hard on my body over the last

year to make sure that I looked perfect in all the pictures we were

going to take. It was important to me to show all my friends across

social media how great we were doing in our new life. I had

swimwear for every day of the week, each with its own funny

image. I couldn't wait to blast these pictures all over the place

from the deck of our ship, next to the bar, double-fisting frozen

cocktails with a cloudless blue sky behind me. Of course I needed

the right angles and the right lighting. Then I would need to use a

filter on the photo to really enhance it and make it pop. My self-

centered head was swelling by the minute. But wasn't this

Alaina's birthday vacation?

Before we could get the kids dropped off, our cruise was

cancelled, 24 hours before we were to set sail. This perfect

vacation that I'd arranged for my wife to include pictures of her

with her new and improved husband with a body to be proud of

collapsed in front of me in a single email.

The Double-Edged Sword

This was not the plan; not my plan. Now what? How was I going to achieve all the "likes" about our vacation now? Alaina did some quick research. We changed our plane ticket from San Juan, Puerto Rico to Miami, Florida. One of Alaina's coworkers who had still been planning to come on the cruise up until the week before had gotten us all a room in San Juan to spend the night before boarding the ship in the morning. Since the cruise was cancelled, she was going to try to join us in Miami and changed the room reservation accordingly. New plan!

For anybody who has never vacationed on a cruise, you pay a fee for your stateroom which includes three meals per day unless you upgrade to a specialty restaurant while on board. You can prepay for an unlimited alcohol package that covers all your drinks over the entire cruise. Unless you are planning to shop at the ports of call or play the casino on the ship, you really don't need much more money once you're aboard.

When you change your plans at the last minute, and go to a beachfront hotel in Miami, it's no longer all-inclusive. So much money had already been invested in the care-free cruise week ahead, but we had our image to uphold. Additionally, I had received a text message from our landlord that there was no rent due for April. We were so grateful for the gesture which increased our vacation budget.

We spent our time on the beach and walking through the shopping district. We would stop at places to have lunch or grab a snack. We even visited a tattoo parlor. Our dinners were only the finest cuisine to be offered. Our third day there was Alaina's birthday. We took to the beach and did the photo shoot we were hoping to do in St. Lucia, but nonetheless had all the props and allure of a proper tropical photo shoot.

The restaurants were closing that night at five. Businesses were closing early. South Beach was already closed, and Spring Break was canceled before we got there. Alaina's birthday dinner consisted of carry-out sushi served in the dining facility inside our hotel lobby. The most gracious concierge provided a complimentary bottle of champagne and plastic flutes. Despite

new restrictions, the night was beautiful.

The next morning we walked to the beach only to find

barricades and caution tape in our path. Our hotel was waiting to

hear if they would be closing. Trailers full of bicycles were going

up and down the streets as the workers were taking apart the bike

rental racks on the sidewalks. Alaina began the process of

changing our flight home. Our vacation was to be cut short.

Ironically, some distance off shore was an anchored cruise

ship running day and night with no noticeable activity aboard. It

was there all week. We later learned the passengers and crew were

quarantined as some people on board were suspected to be positive

with the virus. I hadn't been able to provide the birthday vacation

of my wife's dreams, but she assured me that it was better than

being stuck out there.

The spring of 2020 left us, like many, full of questions.

When we got home we weren't sure if we were going to be able to pick our car up from the airport parking lot because we hadn't heard how Pennsylvania was changing things. We got our car, drove home, and slept. The next morning we went shopping since we had nothing in our house on account of not leaving anything in the refrigerator to spoil while we were away. We had heard about shortages of toilet paper, but seeing it in person was impressive. We gathered what we needed then met with my mother-in-law to retrieve our kids. We returned home to unpack from our travel and from our shopping. Alaina got the message not to come into work until further notice.

In the week that I was away so many emails had been sent out informing us of our own changes in practices. The 911 center had initiated a new protocol for taking calls pertaining to anybody with fever, chest pain, or shortness of breath. I left my home the next day, knowing that I was going in to face this giant head on.

Chapter 9: The battleground

"For I am convinced that neither death nor life, neither angels nor demons, neither the present nor the future, nor any powers, neither height nor depth, nor anything else in all creation, will be able to separate us from the love of God that is in Christ Jesus our Lord." --Romans 8:38-39

Everybody is in masks, including me. The faces that I'd gotten accustomed to seeing around were now partially covered by a paper or material face covering. All the familiar faces were now being upstaged by the most visible piece of this virus. We got

dispatched for our first run on my first day back from vacation.

We arrived at the scene of a patient's house. The

ambulance had already arrived. This was a patient who had been

experiencing some medical event and the noted symptom was

abnormal breathing. The EMTs were donning white Tyvek suits.

They were putting on the accompanying bonnets and boot covers.

Plastic face shields were placed over their faces with a thick, round

N-95 mask covering their noses and mouths. As they were putting

on theirs, we too had to gown up and cover our faces. We were

now set to approach the person behind that door who was in need

of our attention. This attire was just going to be temporary of

course until we learned more about the virus and how to fix it.

With so much information coming in from all angles

including conspiracy theories, it was a scary time. People were

contracting the virus without knowing until weeks later when they

were being admitted to the hospital alone. As far as I was

concerned, every time I left to go to work I had two weeks left to live. Every day that I made it home, I was endangering my family. This was my mentality for the next couple of months. I tried to post videos encouraging other healthcare providers on my friends list, telling them it was just a short thing we had to endure. We'll power through this, I said. The sun will continue to rise, don't worry. Then the peak occurred.

By the time our state hit our peak we had several staff out on leave for having been exposed to Covid-19. The number of patients we were seeing in bad shape had skyrocketed. Some of our applicable airway and respiratory protocols had changed. Additional safety measures were being taken to ensure that a patient shedding the virus would not put us in harm's way.

As the weather got warmer, the infected population seemed to decrease locally, but we had a problem. We live in a beach town, and people now working from home had nothing better to do than go to the beach. Testing was not yet readily available to the public. The people testing positive were the ones who had made it into their doctor's office or a hospital. The local population had been increasing despite a stay-at-home order that was only loosely enforced.

I needed a distraction. I have been on Facebook almost as long as it has been a thing. I had discovered Instagram a couple years ago. The new sensation for 2020 was Tiktok. Hours upon hours had been spent scrolling through people's minute-long videos showing off their Amazon finds, or their dance moves, or worse their summer beach/pool attire. In the palm of my hand I held a portal to every sort of visual stimuli. I was learning new trends, and seeing more *of* people than I needed to. My wife was home with the kids, I was there between work. But slowly I was becoming only physically present.

Most of our friends weren't coming to visit. We couldn't go out and have fun. We were stuck at home, but at least I had the luxury of going to work right? We were all alone together. We were in this together. The only thing we had to unite us all was hearing that we were all having a bad year. That unity didn't last.

The Double-Edged Sword

My social media was flooded. A Minneapolis man had been killed under the knee of a police officer while bystanders recorded the whole thing. This man shouted out so many times, "I can't breathe," but the police officer restraining him maintained the position. The whole nation was outraged. Racial tension soared. During nation-wide protests, fires broke out throughout some neighborhoods, and additional acts of looting and violence ensued. Politicians blamed each other for not doing enough or for doing too much. Fingers were pointed all over the place attaching labels that further divided the already stressed nation. I wanted to hear more. The "news feed" was a constant movie reel in my head. Swimsuits, violence, outrage, cancel culture, likes, comments, trolls, individuals attacking individuals for differences in opinion. On top of everything else that I had suppressed over the years this constant need for my phone in my hand and my constant need to interact consumed me. I had held so much inside that I was ready to implode on myself. At family functions, I was there but absent. At work I was there pushing my own limits, but so much more had been stowed in the background creating a fog. I was unhappy, I was stressed, I was worried, and I was panicking.

At home I was on edge. The slightest thing would trigger an enraged response. I could feel my heart beating out of my chest. Tourists staying in our neighborhood would treat my kids like the plague and warn their children to stay away because they didn't want to get sick. I couldn't lose my temper because next week when they were gone, I still had to live here. I had to hold it all together. Anxiety had set in, turned on the TV, kicked up its feet, and appeared as if it was ready to stay for a long, long time.

Outwardly, I was fine. I'm a paramedic, remember? I am supposed to be helping everybody else during this time. I don't need help. I don't need to talk about the stress to anybody because *everybody* is having a bad year. We're all in this together. I was in control of myself. I had it all under control. My smiles (under my mask) and my motivation had all been manufactured at this point. I still wanted to do the best for my patients. I still wanted to save lives. But I had finally reached the point in my head where I was predicting which patients were taking their last ride with us

and which ones we'd be seeing again soon.

At the end of the spring I had still been working overtime.

When summer came, I backed off. I wanted to preserve whatever

summer was going to be left, and I think it was time off that was

greatly needed. I had signed up for an overtime shift one day in

late May or early June for ten hours that day. We were informed

during our morning conference call that there was a protest

planned for later that day. We have a city within our county that

has had its share of problems, but today they were going to rally

for justice.

We had already seen so many times how these peaceful

protests could take a violent turn. We were optimistic that it

wasn't going to be the case here, but my partner and I both decided

early that if things were to take a turn, we would volunteer to stay

as long as we were needed to keep additional paramedic units

available. By nightfall we were wearing ballistic vests and helmets.

We were positioning ourselves strategically just outside city limits.

Our medic units inside the city were pulled out to also stage

outside the city, ready to respond back in. I started work at eight

that morning and didn't leave for home until two the next morning.

When you watch on the news that things are falling apart in

distant cities, states, and countries, it's a shame. When it happens

that close to home, it hurts so bad. I love this job because it gives

me the opportunity to make a difference in someone's life. It puts

me in a position that at a person's darkest moment they are

reaching out for me. I run into strange houses and businesses to

come face to face with a stranger to help them to start feeling

better if possible or address immediate life threats if necessary.

When all of society is in an uproar, the job doesn't change. The

added stress of the job does. It changes the approach to every

scene. It changes the way you survey your surroundings. It puts in

the forefront that no matter how bad off the person in front of you

is, your goal is to go home at the end of the shift.

A week or so after the protests, my regular partner and I

were dispatched to the scene of a man down. The information

given to us was that a male in his 20s had fallen and hit his head.

When we arrived we saw the EMTs with their stretcher out, trying

to get this man to sit down on it to be assessed. Instead he was

chest to chest against the police officers while onlookers had their

camera phones up in the air recording. My partner was ready to

sedate him, but we hadn't established that he was going to be a

patient yet. For all we knew he may not have wanted us at all. I

was able to talk him into letting us check him out and verify that he

was safe. If he wanted to refuse anything further that would be on

him once we addressed our concerns with him. He relaxed, sat on

the stretcher, and was loaded into the ambulance.

My partner began the assessment. I was connecting the

heart monitor to get blood pressure and heart rate data. Without

warning, he swung a right hook at my partner. She saw it coming

and turned so that her shoulder would take the blow, not her head.

At that point the police assisted us in securing him to the stretcher

in a method safe for transport without him becoming a hazard to himself or others. My partner was very upset with me for not seeing that coming and sedating him sooner.

After that night, the snowball was rolling out of control, but it was totally fine because *I was* in control. Everything was building. The moments of panic increased. There was defeat on my mind every day. With my wife finally back to work, we could plan better for things to come. We spent our money buying stuff to keep us happy while we were instructed to stay at home. Now, all the financial stress was diving head first into the snowball. I was surrounded by my thoughts. The bills were piling up. We made rent by raiding already depleted savings accounts. Investment accounts had been drained. I was being coddled by dancing girls, photos, likes, comments, food trends, life hacks, and now the election season was in full swing. All the hate in the world had surfaced and was being shoved in my face every day from the palm of my hand.

Alaina had been depressed herself, but I was too distracted to notice. I didn't recognize that she felt so alone. Her closest non-work friend was four hours away. A phone call is one thing, but a hug does so much more. She got to see our babysitter, Maggie, regularly, and occasionally we would go out with her and her mom.

By 2020 Maggie had been with us for two years. The sitter we had originally hired to stay at home with the kids began to show a lack of reliability, and there were days that Alaina was walking in late or calling off from work because of childcare. One day she reached out to a local group on Facebook to see if there was anybody who could help or could recommend somebody who could. A man volunteered his homeschooled daughter, and my wife was able to go to work.

The next time we ran into a jam she wasn't available, but her friend was. That girl wasn't available the next time, but Maggie was. This was our girl. When we got home from work, the kids were well cared for. The kitchen was clean; the dining area where the kids ate was clean. We had no mess, including toys to clean up after a long day away. Maggie continued in the position from that day forward. What we didn't know was that each of these girls went to church together and participated in the youth group with Maggie's mother as the youth leader.

As great as Maggie was, I treated her so poorly. I made her feel like she was beneath me and never good enough for us. I didn't know it then, but she had cried to Alaina about me many times. I would throw fits over some of the most nonsensical things.

We already had the youth group watching our kids, so we decided to check out the church. Even with the warm welcome and Maggie's mom by our side, something was missing. A neighbor of ours that we had met at the pool also recommended a different church for us to try. I responded that it was just a miracle that my presence at the first one didn't get me struck by lightning or cause the place to burn down. I wasn't willing to push my luck. We attended Maggie's church as we could but eventually lost the dedication. Then we moved again, 20 minutes away, to another rental closer to our jobs.

The Double-Edged Sword

Alaina felt that she had no friends nearby. I was always glued to my phone. She would talk to me and receive empty responses or noises in return. I wasn't paying close attention. When she would get upset and tell me that I didn't listen to her, she was right. When she told me I always treated her terribly, I would cite things that I had given her or done for her to invalidate her claim that I am *always* treating her poorly. She would tell me that I needed to find counseling and learn how to communicate. I always scoffed at the thought. I did communicate, with all the wrong influences.

In September, Piper began kindergarten. The school bus pulled up. She got out of the car in her first-day-of-school outfit and eagerly approached the bus. I was so wrapped up in trying to get the right pictures to post to social media that I really think I missed the part about my baby growing up too fast. I may have, but our 3-year-old hadn't. The bus pulled away out of sight and he lost it, crying so hard with his face buried in Alaina's shoulder. Alaina told me she was proud of me for not crying. How could I

122

even experience the moment? I was 30 steps ahead, thinking about the content of the profound statement I would post to my life's highlights reel. I have pictures, but was I even there? "Pics, or it didn't happen," right?

The next weekend, we took a trip to go back home and visit friends. Alaina had been telling me about the police officer who helped her through a very rough time in her life. I had met him before, and he had attended our wedding. She was telling me that he was in the hospital possibly having cardiac issues again. She was reading to me from their conversation as well as his posts to Facebook. At that point it had just been a conversation in the car about our friend.

I was already in a mood about going back home because I was now so far above the person I was when I'd lived there, or so I thought. I had a bunch of aspirations of seeing old friends. I had a plan in my head of how the whole weekend would go. I was only up for the 4-day weekend, but Alaina was staying for the week for a wedding.

The Double-Edged Sword

As the weekend progressed I couldn't execute the plans I had laid out. Money was tight. I had our kids while she was helping with wedding stuff. Places I wanted to visit and people I wanted to see were out of reach because of Covid-19 restrictions and being cautious. My old partner came with us to a petting zoo but had clearly gotten over me leaving my old job. She barely spoke to me. She used to be Aunt Brittany to my kids. They didn't remember her.

Among the people I wanted to see was the man that we had resuscitated three years ago. I wanted to catch up with him and his wife, but it was in his best interests not to get sick obviously. The year wasn't just happening to me. I knew this but somehow couldn't accept that things were not the same as the last time I had been up to visit. I was disappointed and angry. I couldn't shake the feeling.

By Monday, Alaina was also angry at me for the way I was acting. I was distant. I wouldn't talk much. I was miserable. I was negative about everything. We had an argument before bed.

She told me once again that I needed to seek counseling. I was still resistant and blew off her statement that obviously had been made out of anger. She told me I needed to figure things out if I thought she was ever coming back home with me. This was the first time she had ever indicated that we might need a break. I went to bed furious. In the morning I woke up extra early and drove two and a half hours to get back to work for my first day shift. I went about my day in my usual fashion. I was fine outwardly. Inside, not so much.

I got home that night and had been carrying on small talk with Alaina on the phone. I kept hearing a sound like my phone was sending me notifications, but I was on my phone. I told her about it to have her help me figure out what it could be. Not being home with me, she didn't hear it and really I couldn't expect her to itemize everything in our house to pinpoint my *current* annoyance since *everything* apparently annoyed me.

As the night progressed I kept hearing it intermittently, not enough to rely on the sound to lead me to the source, although I had gotten closer than I knew at one point using this method until it stopped again. At bedtime I got in our king size bed alone, set my alarms for the morning, and attempted to close my eyes. Then it happened again.

On the dresser across from the foot of our bed was our laptop. I opened it. My wife had been logged onto her Facebook account, and the messenger component was chiming every time a message was received. There was a group chat displayed for a business group my wife was involved with, and there must've been a hot topic that night because there were so many messages being exchanged, the source of the sound. Also displayed was another conversation window with the police officer that we had been discussing earlier in the weekend. I read one message out of context that set me on fire. It set the tone for everything else that I ended up reading back through. It was a very short conversation that had spanned several years. Like me and *my* friends, there were long periods of time between short conversations. I didn't recognize that though because my rage had taken over.

The way I read this thing was like a secret plot on the side. I projected my previous promiscuous ways onto them. I was way over my head and suddenly drowning in every emotion, unable to control myself. I couldn't call her and ask her what this was because she would think I was intentionally spying on her. I wasn't. I was chasing the messaging app tone. This was just the icing on the cake. If they were plotting something and I called her then I would stop it from happening. If it were to happen and I asked her about it later, would she lie to me? Lie to me? There hadn't been a day in our life that I didn't trust Alaina. What was happening? Seeing the conversation with my added assumptions was like pulling the flush handle, and now there I was, circling the drain.

At that moment, my life choices caught up with me. I had been a terrible person for so long before Alaina and I began our relationship. I was juggling women like a street performer juggles batons on fire. I had been the guy the wife snuck off to. I had been suggestive to more married women who didn't return the advances. I was the guy that had two women I was fooling around with, meeting me at the same bar at the same time to literally compete for my attention and buy me drinks, only to get up and walk out on both of them without offering to pay for anything. More than anything, I absolutely deserved what I had coming to me.

At that point I realized that I did in fact need help. As I saw it, my marriage was on thin ice, but of course *I* wasn't the heat source. I sent a text message to Maggie's mom, the youth pastor, and begged for advice, wisdom, a solution, anything. It was late at night. She also worked. She wasn't awake. I lay on my bed and stared at the ceiling, enraged until I fell asleep.

When I got to work in the morning, my partner saw I was sluggish. She drove me to get coffee. Even after reaching the bottom of the cup, I was no better. We talked all day about what I had seen, and she tried so hard to work through it with me. Unfortunately at one point she validated my concern, and I was in the deepest, darkest place I had ever known. So now what? We talked it out and decided that I would leave work that night and drive back up to Alaina, all 2 and a half hours. If in fact I had driven her into the company of another man, chances were I would know by the end of the night. At any rate we needed to talk. I had left things in a very bad way.

By the afternoon I had received a response from Maggie's mom. She texted me a name and phone number of a counselor she knew of and told me to call. I reached out, and we set up a Zoom conference 2 weeks later. At the end of that shift, my partner was taking leave for surgery. This was only our second day shift; I had two night shifts ahead. Who was I going to talk to now? Whatever random partner showed up tomorrow night? No. I had to put on a show for them. I was bulletproof and there to save the world.

Just before the end of my shift I got a phone call from my platoon commander. He told me he heard my voice on the radio throughout the day, and that everybody was worried about me. He told me he wasn't prying but wanted me to know that although he was my supervisor he would also let me talk and hold it in confidence. He offered to help in any way that he could.

"No, sir. I'm just a little bummed about something right now. I'm good." I just kept digging my hole deeper.

At the end of the day, I had to say goodbye to my partner as she was going to be out for a while. With a stern tone, she instructed me not to do anything stupid. She reassured me I could let her know what happened, but not late at night.

Alaina called me when I was in my car and on my way. I hadn't told her what I was doing. I was making the trek and we did some talking. Soon she realized that I had not gotten home yet. She asked me where I was. I told her I was on the road, almost there (meaning home).

"Almost where?" she asked.

"To you," I sheepishly responded.

She already knew. She could hear something different about my voice, and my phone service was cutting out more often than the two poor spots I ordinarily drove through. She sounded excited that I was coming back. But she also confirmed I was doing this because I wanted to. I'd made it clear before I left that I didn't want to return for a very long time. She waited up for my arrival, and when I got there I was very well received. I spent most of the next day with her and informed her that I had a scheduled appointment with a counselor. She seemed so relieved that I had finally reached out to somebody for help. I needed it, especially because I could not bring myself to engage her in conversation about the messages I saw.

Chapter 10: Bandaging the wounds

"Is anyone among you sick? Let him call for the elders of the

church, and let them pray over him, anointing him with oil in the

name of the Lord. And the prayer of faith will save the one who is

sick, and the Lord will raise him up. And if he has committed sins,

he will be forgiven. Therefore, confess your sins to one another

and pray for one another, that you may be healed. The prayer of a

righteous person has great power as it is working." --James 5:14-

16

The most successful business of the year 2020 almost has to be the owners of the Zoom software. I had learned that my appointment with the therapist would be done via Zoom. I had not had the privilege of using Zoom at all during the course of the pandemic as so many had, so now I had the added stress of figuring out how all of that worked. Since I didn't have to leave my house for the meeting, I had the additional anxiety that if Alaina didn't have to work she would be able to hear everything. Her schedule worked out favorably, so the only challenge was remembering to get on the app on time.

There I sat with my earbuds in place and the meeting screen in front of me. I was waiting for the host to let me into the meeting. I knew nothing about her except her name. I hadn't researched reviews or anything. If she was the recommendation of the youth minister, she had to be good, right? But what if she wasn't? A face appeared in front of me and began talking. First we set some ground rules, then we launched.

The most important thing to know about counseling is that you need to be completely open and honest. I was tired. I was done feeling like I was. I wanted my wife to be happy again. I wanted to be able to function again. So when she asked how she could help, I unloaded.

"Are you a Christian?" she asked.

So many times this question has come up. Every time it was the same response. When I confirmed that I was, she informed me that she would incorporate biblical references into our time together. Great, I thought. You're not going to be able to help me, so you are going to bring God into this to make it all better. Fantastic. Got it.

I explained everything that had taken place on our trip. I opened up and dumped my story in her lap to sort through. She sat there calmly looking concerned and began to help me sort through the pieces bit by bit. As I was talking there were notifications popping up about text messages coming from the therapist. What was this?

As we sorted through the mess that I had laid out for her she made reference to different podcasts and told me she'd already sent the links. In our weekly meetings she would help me categorize the information and would refer to each piece with practical guidance. She wasn't beating me in the head with the Bible. She was passing me media to read or listen to or watch. My commute to and from work allowed me to listen to the podcasts in the privacy of my own car. I hadn't discussed with Alaina anything the therapist and I had talked about, especially figuring out how to tell Alaina I had read those messages.

We talked about my financial stress, my stress in the family, my mood swings, my general negative attitude. She had pointed me in the direction of a well-known pastor and Christian author who had written several books that she thought might help guide me. I had already been listening to audiobooks that were self-help for negative thinking and self-help for personal financial freedom. I was listening to books written by politicians and I listened to one book dramatized out of the horror genre. I was already listening to audiobooks, so what was I changing by listening to *these* podcasts and audiobooks she was recommending?

I did Catholic school from 6th to 9th grade. I had my own Bible. We would refer to it, and highlight required verses. I loved going to church on Fridays because the rest of my classes the rest of the day were shortened to get them all in with the added time it took for church. I had done the Bible thing and the church thing, but I still felt how I felt at this point. What were we solving?

So I listened to the podcast. The pastor on the podcast was the same one that had authored the book I was to listen to. When I wasn't in my car, I had started journaling and would take notes while listening to the books on audio. I would have a bad day and start dumping it out into the journal. I was getting my feelings out on paper and not suppressing them. I was writing them down where they could be mine, and I didn't have to worry about anybody getting a hold of them. I was embarrassed to be in this position, seeking help and writing down my feelings, but I soon found out I didn't have to be. What I was doing was beginning to help. I wasn't carrying the weight of an argument around to fester and build inside me. I was occupying my time with writing about everything that was hurting me and stressing me out. If I yelled at the kids, it was in there. If Alaina and I had a spat, it was in there.

I had been hearing about individuals in the Bible facing their own struggles. I had found out how they overcame them. In some cases, there were supernatural occurrences which I didn't care to hear, but in other ways they held onto teachings that had been there all their lives and remembered what was said and held onto so many promises and so much wisdom. They figured out their way through some divine inspiration. One book I listened to referred specifically to marriage and how we take these vows and at the end say "so help me God " like it's just another oath swearing us in to some legal obligation. Even Alaina and I invested so much time planning our perfect wedding day, but we didn't have a plan for the next morning, week, year, etc. So this book would be a guide to make that plan. The knowledge shared was straight out of the Bible.

After several audiobooks and podcasts, I learned a few lessons. If a pack of wolves sees a lone wolf, they take it into their pack and foster it because wolves are pack hunters and their best chance of survival is their strength in numbers. Nobody struggling in the Bible got there all at once; there was a progression to their arrival in their predicament. So if these authors were able to regurgitate this information for me using the Bible as reference, maybe I too should read the Bible. If I kept answering the question in the affirmative that I was in fact a Christian, perhaps I should actually research what I was agreeing to.

It didn't take long for news of my counseling to travel. My in-laws were present for my kids' autumn birthday parties. My father-in-law, who I had sought advice from in the past and who had tried to pull me closer to his faith, took the opportunity to ask me how I was doing.

For somebody with an ego problem like I had, when somebody asks you how counseling is going, it's like standing in front of them completely naked, stripped of any cloak you've been hiding under. The question was up in the air, out in the open. As physics teaches us, what goes up must come down. You better have an answer. Will it be the right answer? It's fine. Ugh!!!!! Back at this again? *That* was the answer I had for my father-in-law? So frustrating!

Then he asked me if my therapist was a spiritual counselor. Why yes she is; Christian, too.

"Do you know him?"

"I was referred to her by a friend, and we have already been meeting for a month or so, so yeah I guess I know her. Her husband is a pastor."

"No. Do you know Him?" he asked as he pointed upward. "God."

The Double-Edged Sword

Now this was a great question. I got really excited to tell him what I had been learning, but at the same time I didn't want to offend him if my learnings didn't align with his much more strict Catholic background.

"I honestly didn't. But I am learning so much."

One nice thing Alaina and I have had throughout our marriage is a very loose Christian faith. Between online movie streaming services and her parents, we would get some really good recommendations for movies to watch. When we would come across a religious movie, we would try it out. The movies were often based on somebody's true life experience and dramatized by big name actors, whether Hollywood A-listers or main line Christian actors. We had seen a child's near-death experience reveal what Heaven might be like. We had seen a college freshman defend the existence of God. One night we were watching a movie about a singer who joined a band and wrote a song. At the end of the movie, when I heard the song and recognized it from so many years ago, I was shocked. I hadn't

realized until then the inspirational story behind that singer.

Between the podcasts and books I was now listening to,

and the movies we had seen, I had a loose mosaic of what God was

like. But how did we get here? Why do so many people blindly

follow this faith in hope of something so great at the end? I am a

paramedic. I know what happens at the end. I write the time the

person was pronounced on a tag with an incident number that

becomes their identity to the medical examiner, if he is to be

involved. So why are so many people so drawn in? And why are

there so many people so skeptical to the same point?

In one of our sessions, I told my therapist that I had learned

about the wolves. I found it to be an intriguing analogy because

more often I had heard Christians referred to as sheep by a blind

society. But the point of the wolves story is that if you try to take

on Christianity alone, you will be lost. The best way to understand

where you fit is to find your church and let the wolf pack take you

in. But we'd tried that.

The Double-Edged Sword

Back home Alaina would attend a church with her best friend when she had the day off and while I was at work. The kids would go to a kids room, and Alaina seemed to enjoy herself there. I attended once with them. We tried to go to Maggie's church, but it didn't do it for me. Then I remembered our neighbors from the pool. They had plugged their church in a conversation and mentioned it was a young, fun crowd.

The next Sunday I worked I decided to explore churches. When I uncovered their church and found my way to the Facebook page, I saw that they were live streaming the Sunday service. I watched the live service and realized that I hadn't put my phone down or drifted off to another activity. When the service was over I did more research, a website. They had a location two miles from our home. I watched a video of a previous live stream. Was this church? It had to be. They were talking about Jesus. They were singing. The band was really good, and the people were into it, hands in the air and everything, just like on TV. And I had learned that they were holding in person services now with a close compliance to the pandemic guidelines. I would have to reserve my seat ahead of time.

The next Sunday that I had off, Alaina worked, and I had the kids. So I signed the kids up for kids' church, and I saved myself a seat. There weren't many in attendance in person, and we all had our masks on. We were seated with distance in mind. The following Wednesday was Veterans Day, so the service opened up by asking all the veterans to stand. I stood with a few other people, and an usher walked up to me with a dozen glazed donuts in a box. He thanked me for my service and told me to enjoy some donuts on them. What? The band took the stage, and this room became electric. I was expecting to come to church and hear some hymns, but this was a rock concert for Christ. The last song slowed down and the lead singer said a prayer before telling everyone to sit. The pastor took the stage and called up the director of one of the services offered by the church. This young man had just turned 30 and had received his ordination as a minister. The pastor said a few kind, insightful words and then congratulated him. The pastor was beginning the last sermon of a multi-week series. He was a young guy, mid to late 30s himself. He was very hyper and convicted and charismatic. I sat there and listened to him speak for the time he had with us, and I was impressed by his message.

Not only was the content relevant, but the way he presented it was relevant, too. He himself recognized that he is human, imperfect in this imperfect world. He wasn't preaching from atop his own ivory soapbox. He wasn't chastising us for our flaws. He was telling us about his own moments of imperfection and also making reference to Mountain Dew. For the length of the service I sat there intently, listening to everything he had to say, and when he was done, he prayed over us. After the prayer he informed us that a new series would start next week called "Family Matters," and if we had kids in the kids' church to sit down and relax as our kids would be brought in to us.

Afterward, the pastor made his way to the back of the room and told me he had never seen me there before. I introduced myself and told him I was a little star struck after watching him for the last couple weeks on Facebook. We chatted for a short couple of minutes before my kids ran up to me, excited to tell me about their experience. At the moment I didn't understand how such a strange place to me and even to the kids could feel so familiar. And how had I found my way inside just in time to start a series about family matters, the focus of my therapy? What a coincidence, right?

Alaina joined me the following week as we embarked on this journey of family struggles. We listened closely as the pastor shared stories of parenting, struggles in his own marriage, the same little arguments everybody has. The stories were funny because they were true. They were relevant. It didn't feel the way that I knew church felt previously. People yelled out "Amen" when a point spoke to them. The pastor was calling people out by first name. There was laughter. There was joy. There was peace. There was Alaina sitting next to me, she herself engaged in the message. We had found our church, our wolf pack.

The Double-Edged Sword

We had been in such a terrible place. Our finances were out of alignment, and our priorities too. We couldn't agree on anything but to disagree. We told each other every day that we loved each other. That was fact, and it hadn't changed. What had changed was whether we were capable of wholly believing each other in those moments. I love you, but I'm not in love with you. I love you, but I don't like you right now. It's not you, it's me. These clichés were paving the path we had been heading down. But here we were in this new place together. It wasn't strange. I walked in feeling like I was right where I belonged. Alaina concurred with my assessment. Finally, we had taken a step in the right direction, and we had done it together.

In my next therapy session, we discussed my experiences and shared in the joy of finding a church to attend. The podcasts and books were great, but to be in person with other people of similar age with similar life struggles, was much more rewarding and impactful. The therapist congratulated me and assured me I was getting back on the right track.

"Jesus continued: "There was a man who had two sons.

The younger one said to his father, 'Father, give me my share of

the estate.' So he divided his property between them. Not long

after that, the younger son got together all he had, set off for a

distant country and there squandered his wealth in wild living.

After he had spent everything, there was a severe famine in that

whole country, and he began to be in need. So he went and hired

himself out to a citizen of that country, who sent him to his fields

to feed pigs. He longed to fill his stomach with the pods that the

pigs were eating, but no one gave him anything. When he came to

his senses, he said, 'How many of my father's hired servants have

food to spare, and here I am starving to death! I will set out and go

back to my father and say to him: Father, I have sinned against

heaven and against you. I am no longer worthy to be called your

son; make me like one of your hired servants.' So he got up and

went to his father. But while he was still a long way off, his father

saw him and was filled with compassion for him; he ran to his son,

threw his arms around him and kissed him. The son said to him,

'Father, I have sinned against heaven and against you. I am no longer worthy to be called your son.' But the father said to his servants, 'Quick! Bring the best robe and put it on him. Put a ring on his finger and sandals on his feet. Bring the fattened calf and kill it. Let's have a feast and celebrate. For this son of mine was dead and is alive again; he was lost and is found.' So they began to celebrate. Meanwhile, the older son was in the field. When he came near the house, he heard music and dancing. So he called one of the servants and asked him what was going on. 'Your brother has come,' he replied, 'and your father has killed the fattened calf because he has him back safe and sound.' The older brother became angry and refused to go in. So his father went out and pleaded with him. But he answered his father, 'Look! All these years I've been slaving for you and never disobeyed your orders. Yet you never gave me even a young goat so I could celebrate with my friends. But when this son of yours who has squandered your property with prostitutes comes home, you kill the fattened calf for him!' 'My son,' the father said, 'you are always with me, and everything I have is yours. But we had to celebrate and be glad,

because this brother of yours was dead and is alive again; he was

lost and is found.'" -- Luke 15: 11-32

Chapter 11: Healing the pain

My days were full of self-reassurance. I was no longer waking up angry that I had made it through the night. I was able to start my day with a short, quick motto and set my own mood without my mood dictating my day. I had been waking up angry. Alaina knew on those days, the majority of them, I was not going to be pleasant to be around and I was a ticking time bomb. But something was different. I knew how hard I was trying. I knew that I needed to explain myself sometimes, but I couldn't expect my family to read my mind. That had failed miserably time after time.

Instead of erupting at my kids for leaving something on the floor, I would simply ask them if they like nice Daddy or mean Daddy. They always tell me they like nice Daddy. They are so much more compliant to my requests when I remind them that there is a difference between the two. The fact that they recognized the difference between nice Daddy and mean Daddy is profound. I had learned through my counseling that God gave me the family intended for me and entrusted me to lead them, ultimately to Him. So when mean Daddy would overpower and speak sharply, chastising, berating, angry, I was failing to lead. My focus had changed from the things around me influencing my attitude to being focused on God and reflecting his leadership on the things around me.

To heal myself, I had to come clean to Alaina. We had been discussing homes and getting a mortgage. Any homeowner knows this is a huge commitment. I took the conversation as an

opportunity to transition into my confession. I told her if we were

going to take this step, I need to be sure that it is 100% me and her.

She assured me it was. I repeated myself. Concerned, she restated

that it is. When I said it the third time, she asked me why wouldn't

it be?

I asked her to think back to September, when we made the

trip home, and the night after I left to go to work. I was talking on

the phone with her and had asked her about the sound. She didn't

remember. I went on to explain that when I went to bed I heard it

again. I told her I opened up the laptop and saw her business

group chat full of new, unread messages; but I also saw her

conversation with our friend that hurt me so badly. I told her that I

was very confused and upset by the conversation. I told her that it

looked like she was trying to convince him to go along as her

wedding date. He was leaving for Florida and couldn't attend the

wedding. Since he couldn't make it, it appeared they were trying

to plan something else, but nothing materialized. I told her I was hurt that she hadn't said anything to me about asking him to be her wedding date. I couldn't attend because of work, but having read as far back as I did it looked like the last wedding they went to was much more than a friendly encounter. There were also messages from a woman who sent them through the police officer's social media account, a woman who he was having an affair with while also cheating on his wife with Alaina.

Alaina explained that despite my invitations to him to visit us at the beach, he did not want to feel like he was making me uncomfortable by their past relationship. She stressed that he respected me. Then she asked me why I felt like that was even a possibility for her. She had never given me any reason not to trust her. She had been nothing but faithful and by my side since the beginning, as was I.

I explained that I had been in a terrible place because of how I left things when I left her to go to work. I told her that I was afraid that I had done that much damage to drive her to him. She reassured me that was not the case. He had been invited to the wedding by the bride, and she hadn't seen him since our wedding. She said their conversations have always had a flirty tone but she'd tone it down or not continue their friendship if that was what I wanted.

That wasn't fair. I would never ask her to terminate a friendship. His role in her life went beyond anything romantic. During a terrible time in her life, he'd kept her alive. In much the same way, I've had conversations with long-time female friends that may have also had a flirtatious tone. When this is how we communicate for years, it may be hard to just turn it off. Besides, I wasn't exactly holding my own in our relationship either.

Social media was a great tool for staying in touch with friends I'd been deployed with, and family, and friends from elementary school, and so forth. But it came at a cost. Enticing ads were displayed for apps of a pornographic nature. I was adding female friends over time. When they would go on vacation

to a tropical destination, I couldn't help checking out their pictures.
I was drawn in and glued. I would scroll my news feed and see
more and more things like this that would just suck me in.

When TikTok gained popularity, I would see videos and
give them a like. Then TikTok would give me more videos of a
similar nature. Before too long, all I was seeing was girls pole
dancing and dancing in swimwear that didn't leave much to the
imagination. I was a fish hooked by a pro angler. Don't get me
wrong; it wasn't all temptation.

Connecting with others sometimes offered great little catch
phrases or words to live by. "A beautiful day starts with a
beautiful mindset." This spoke to me when I needed it most. But
the problem was the stuff I didn't need. I was also trapped in
every political post, watching people just tear each other apart
about their own opinions. People would watch videos they had no
interest in just to insert their own political agendas into the

comments and start fights from the comfort of their keyboard.

Hate was spewing from everywhere.

If this wasn't enough, all of my interests that I had shared over the years were in front of me in the form of ads beckoning me on my next cruise, showing me everyone else's perfect lives doing the activities that I would enjoy doing. And finally, anything I spoke about was connected to some sort of merchandising ad.

When I found my way into counseling and started praying out loud over meals and discovering my prayer life, I had ads for apparel identifying me as a pastor. It was enough. One by one I got rid of the social machine and all the agendas that had been keeping me from living my life. I finally rediscovered how much fun it was to get on the floor with my kids or run around outside with them. Our time spent together was more than me camping on the couch with my phone in my hand, separating me from the rest of my life.

Chapter 12: A Spirit Revived

Getting back to my father-in-law's question a couple chapters ago, do I know God? Still no, but I'm getting closer. I have received so much information and guidance from my therapist and pastor. On my first day visiting the church, I left with a new coffee cup, a dozen glazed donuts, and a Bible. So here I was with this resource in front of me, in my possession. I vowed on our wedding day to lead our family with Christ preeminent; but I didn't know what that meant. So like anything

else you want to know more about, you research.

Genesis chapter 1, verse 1: "In the beginning God created

the heavens and the earth." If I wanted to learn about God, this

seemed like a great place to start. As I continued to read I was

rediscovering stories that I already knew, some that I had never

heard, and clarifying some of the stories that were told in a way to

ease the message to a child so many years ago. What I learned was

that the people in this book whom God chose to speak through and

to perform His works were by no means idols to look up to when

he found them. Adam and Eve were given everything they needed

by God, but when they were tempted by more they gave in to the

temptation. Noah was a drunk, but he was selected to help God

wipe out and repopulate the world. Moses was a murderer, as were

many other figures we have heard of in our lifetime.

I had been told that the easiest way to read the Bible was to

find a reading plan that takes chunks from all over the Bible and puts them together with a common theme. You could usually find these and complete the whole Bible in a year. I already had such a scattered impression of Christianity. I was already scattered in my thoughts and my emotions. I was not willing to learn God in pieces. Instead I took the Bible and read it straight through as the world history textbook that it is. If you want to learn about the wrath of God, read the Old Testament. When God was scorned he delivered consequences. He laid out the law to Moses on top of a mountain, but the people remained skeptical of their purpose. As time went on God was making and keeping promises. He was protecting his people like his own children. By the end of the Old Testament people were out in the marketplaces and temples telling everybody, if you think this is good, the best is yet to come.

When I got to the New Testament, I had been told by my mother-in-law and my therapist to download an app on my phone and watch this series about Jesus. In the car, I was reading about the life and works of Jesus. With friends and family, I was watching this app-based series that took the words off the page and painted Jesus in a new perspective. At the end of the first season, I was devastated. I wanted to see more. I was invested now.

I started Genesis on Thanksgiving and set the goal to go cover to cover by New Year's Eve. Even my therapist thought that was ambitious. She recommended that I read the Old Testament in that period of time and start the new year with the New Testament. I fell short of my goal, but by the second week of January I completed Revelation. For the first time in my life, I had read the Bible. My whole life I was of the Christian faith, but I didn't know how deep Christianity was until I read. It's not an easy task to complete. It takes steadfast dedication. You have to plan your time to sit and read and to listen to it in audio form. You can do it. Believe me, if I can, you can.

Did reading the Bible turn me into an overnight evangelist? No. Simply stated, it gave me a foundation to build my life on. I was created by a loving, almighty Father who is the same today as He was yesterday and always will be. His hand created Heaven and Earth. He painted the stars to His liking. He created man in His image and gave us free will. He provides everything we *need* as long as we are willing to ask. He doesn't ask us for much but to love Him first and then love others.

What kind of love is this? Even while we were still sinning against the Father in Heaven, God sent his Son down from Heaven to be born of a virgin, to teach, to make his presence known, and then to suffer publicly before dying to conquer death and save us from our sins. Everybody on Calvary watched as the Son of God took his last breath, gave up His spirit, and His flesh died on the cross. He was placed into a sealed tomb with guards. Amidst all of this He got up three days later and walked among the same people who both loved Him and those who hated Him. He revealed to the world who God was because he embodied God.

I accept Jesus Christ as my Lord and Savior, and I will honor the man that He was and honor God, whom He is. I will choose to love others. Our time on this Earth is short, too short it

161

feels. But if I walk guided by the Holy Spirit that was, is, and always will be, I can lead my family home to Heaven when God is ready to bring us home. Through God, the Father, the Son, and the Holy Spirit, we have victory over death. Our spirits live on eternally after our bodies fail.

So if this is true, and I believe whole-heartedly that it is, then when I get into the back of the ambulance with a patient in some form of physical crisis, I know that I have more than a cluster of cells and tissues in front of me. I have a son or daughter of our Heavenly Father, my brother or sister in Christ. They themself may not know it. God gave everybody free will. God gives us faith, hope, and love. He has assured us that temptation is not from Him. I can treat this patient's ailment, and sometimes there will be victory, sometimes not. But if we treat the person's spirit as well, I am certain that we will win every time.

This doesn't mean that I am going to preach the whole way to the hospital; I have a job to do. But if everything I have learned and everything that I have read are accurate, shouldn't sharing

God's love be enough? Regardless of where the patient is at in

their own spirituality, they can recognize love. It's natural. Since

God is love, I can bring Him to them just by showing love.

Babies love naturally. They grow in their mother's womb

receiving nourishment. They're born and know who their mother

is. Their spirit, though, has been loved by God for so long before

that they already know what love is. Anything other than love is

taught by experiences, choices, and being of the world. I have

learned that although I am *in* the world, I am not *of* the world.

I am one of God's chosen. The same God that caused a big

bang (Science says energy can be neither created nor destroyed,

only transferred) and painted the universe, and created everything

in it, also created me; and before I was born into this world, He

already knew my name. And He knew you. He knows you. He

hasn't changed. He never will.

The Double-Edged Sword

I have spent years lost to my own interests, my own plans, my own motives, my own doings. I followed the attractive, popular, exciting options; and I forgot what love was. Love is more than the emotional connection or the butterflies. Love is more than the physical activities behind closed doors. To know love is to know God. No God, no love, right? Know God, know peace, yes? We've seen all the bumper stickers. We've heard the clichés. We've heard the stories. So how do we act?

"God so loved the world that he gave his one and only Son, that whoever believes in him shall not perish but have eternal life." -- John 3:16

Who are you willing to die for? What are you willing to die for? Are you really so consumed in your work and your ego that you bury all your concerns, regrets, emotions, and secrets deep inside you until you have become so consumed by them that all you can do is consume substance? Are you willing to drive yourself to the point that one bad choice leads to another to another and the only way out of facing the consequences is to terminate

your life on *your* own terms?

If you're feeling alone, weak, desperate, overwhelmed,

afraid, or at the end of your rope, it's okay. God sees it. He

already knows. If you want peace, just ask for it; but remember it

comes down to His will, not your own. If you're feeling this way

and you're not ready to face God and talk, then why expedite the

meeting by ending your life? If you're not here yet and unable to

reach up to God and place your worries in His hands, then reach

out to a friend, a coworker, a family member, even a counselor.

If you've never been in this place and you are satisfied in

your life, remember to thank God for your blessings. Be the

person to help the person in need. Don't focus on the labels or

classification or dividers that society has laid out for people. God

sees us plain. Jesus made it clear to love your neighbor as

yourself, as God has loved you. How do you know who your

neighbor is? Go back to chapter one and read the introduction.

Which one of these men was a neighbor to the man?

When He was on trial and made to defend His words, the teachers of the day set Jesus up to commit sin. They asked Him of all the laws that God has given, which of these is the most important? When He responded that the greatest commandment is to love your neighbor, they were taken back. If you simply act with God's love towards everybody you come in contact with, wouldn't the Ten Commandments be fulfilled? So Jesus' point was just love, and you won't end up on the wrong side of the law.

If it's this simple, why isn't everybody a Christian? Why is church attendance down nationwide? Is it because there is some myth that Christians are just sheep that use God as a crutch? It's not a myth. We are sheep, and you should meet our shepherd. When the wolves are coming for us we can look to Him for protection and wisdom. The wolves could be financial, personal, professional, whatever. My God is greater. Do I use God as a crutch? Of course. I *am* weak. I get my strength through God. Physical strength is pointless if you don't have the spirit to control it.

So consider my earlier question. Who are *you* willing to die for? Is there a person you love so much that you would lay your life on the line for them? What if they aren't willing to do the same for you? Would it still be worth it? It *is* possible to love somebody so much without them loving you in return. Divorce, affairs, and abandonment are all real things. You give and give and give without getting in return. Instead they turn on you; they spit in your face. How do you make somebody love you back who you have never stopped loving? It's a great question. Ask Jesus.

For those of us in emergency services, we drop everything and rush to a person having a crisis. We negotiate traffic obstacles. We safely navigate from station to destination, but we can't control the people around us. We could be involved in a crash, we could get hit by a vehicle when we're operating on the highway, we could be attacked by a rogue person when we are trying to help

their first victim. If we're so willing to give our life for a stranger,

isn't that love? We care for their outcome and strive to do the best

possible thing for them. We are already capable of love, so why

not perfect it? If your patient assessment is lacking, don't you lean

on somebody to help perfect it? Then why not lean on God to help

you perfect your love, to take some of the pressure off of you, to

keep you present in the moment, to give you wisdom? Have you

ever prayed with a patient? I have. Have you ever taken a knee

and just thanked God for getting you in and out of the burning

house safely? There's a concept. Have you ever thanked God?

Something great happened or you didn't get picked for a task you

didn't want to do. Did you say, "Thank God!!!"?

If you're already telling Him thank you, couldn't you just

as easily ask for grace? Mercy?

"God, be with this patient as she goes into an unfamiliar

setting. You are the ultimate healer and You already know the cure. Just be with the doctors, and give them the wisdom to find

the problem and to fix it according to Your will. Amen." It's not

hard. It can be short and simple. Prayers are powerful. If you

don't ask, the answer is always no.

Chapter 13: Perspective

How long had I struggled? How long did I offer excuses for everything? My favorite expression from the Army is "the maximum effective range of an excuse is 0 meters," but I spent plenty of time making excuses. How many times had I thought I was at the end? And yet to date I have survived every day of my life. I was drowning, but my head was above water. How?

We long for resources and explanations. We want a degree on the wall, so we read and research. We want to be better parents and spouses, but where's the official textbook for that? The following is a hint where the information can be found:

"Now concerning the matters about which you wrote: "It is good for a man not to have sexual relations with a woman." But because of the temptation to sexual immorality, each man should have his own wife and each woman her own husband. The husband should give to his wife her conjugal rights, and likewise the wife to her husband. For the wife does not have authority over her own body, but the husband does. Likewise the husband does not have authority over his own body, but the wife does. Do not deprive one another, except perhaps by agreement for a limited time, that you may devote yourselves to prayer; but then come together again, so that Satan may not tempt you because of your lack of self-control." 1 Corinthians 7:1-40.   Have a healthy sex life. Any argument?

"Husbands, love your wives, and do not be harsh with them." Colossians 3:19. Show God's love; His grace and His mercy. Don't rule your house by your hand.

171

The Double-Edged Sword

"Husbands, love your wives, as Christ loved the church and gave himself up for her, that he might sanctify her, having cleansed her by the washing of water with the word, so that he might present the church to himself in splendor, without spot or wrinkle or any such thing, that she might be holy and without blemish. In the same way husbands should love their wives as their own bodies. He who loves his wife loves himself. For no one ever hated his own flesh, but nourishes and cherishes it, just as Christ does the church," Ephesians 5:25-35. You say, "I do" as does your spouse. At that moment, with God and others as your witness, you are bound for life until death do us part as one body. As the Spice Girls so eloquently stated in the 90s, "Tonight is the night when two become one." I've learned that this isn't long enough. I want to help my wife get to Heaven so that we can be reunited and continue our eternal life together.

"Be angry and do not sin; do not let the sun go down on your anger, and give no opportunity to the devil." Ephesians 4:26-27. How often do we do this? The argument silences our supper.

We don't talk, call, or text to come to a final resolution. We lay down angry knowing that the last words we spoke could be the last opportunity we have to speak.

"For everyone who exalts himself will be humbled, and he who humbles himself will be exalted." Luke 14:11. You may have the right answer, you may be right in the quarrel. Would you rather stress your point and beat a dead horse continuing to break down your life partner or would you rather agree to disagree? It's more important to love than to be right.

These are just a few passages that give us a foundation to build on. How can they help you if you don't know where to look for them? My relationship suffered. It suffered so bad. It suffered because I allowed myself to walk down a path that wasn't for me. One step at a time, I got further and further from where I needed to be. I didn't go to sleep in the best shape of my life and wake up thinking my marriage was in trouble. It happened one step at a time.

The Double-Edged Sword

"Do not be anxious about anything, but in everything by prayer and supplication with thanksgiving let your requests be made known to God." Philippians 4:6. Thank God that you made it out of the fire. Pray for peace for losses you may have suffered. Thank God for the wisdom to keep up with the demands of the critical patient; but if they weren't yours to save, ask for peace.

"God, you know the work that I do. You know the challenges I'm presented with. I ask that you keep me humble in my duties and wise to execute my duties effectively. Put me where you need me most but soften my heart so that I address the whole need. Give me the strength to fulfill your plan for my life. Thank you for allowing me to serve you in this way you have called me to. In Jesus' name, Amen."

This chapter is very heavy with scripture. Is it uncomfortable? I accept that it might be. I know it used to be for me. My turn to Jesus took a lot of heartache. I needed to turn myself down and turn up the Holy Spirit in myself. I needed to do my own research on Him. I'm happy to report that He is still here doing great work. Just look around.

Human nature and worldly teachings have taught us not to take no for an answer and to hide the truth to avoid the consequences. So often we hear that the laws of God are greater than the laws of men. Accepting Christ means understanding that there are consequences for your actions. Your eternity is on the line. You can't hide from God. He doesn't see as your neighbor sees. He sees what's inside. He already knows your needs, feelings, and desires. He is simply waiting for you to ask for them. Sometimes the answer *is* no. And that is okay.

I would love to take my kids to Disney World because they are old enough to appreciate the experience. I want to take them before they are too cool to react to Mickey or flex with Gaston. I ask God to help me provide for my family. Disney is my plan. It may not be His plan. If I pray for Disney, the answer may be no every time. If I pray for a vacation, the answer still might be no, but if I ask Him to help me provide for my family, He is going to

help me do *that* according to His plan.

Chapter 14: Moving Forward

After reading through my experience, I hope first and foremost that I have not dissuaded somebody from taking a job in the emergency services. It *is* a very rewarding career. It can be very exciting, but you can't make a false idol of it.

For the medic on the street that has read this, think about how I fell down. I pushed and pushed and abused my own adrenaline like a drug. But like all drugs, over time it builds up tolerance. You need more. No, you don't need more of the adrenaline. You need something else in your life that brings you joy. You need to network with people who will support you. And when you've had enough, you need to recognize it and take a break.

Managers, love your people. They were gifted to you by God to help support you. Support them in return. Talk to them. Get to know them. See them for who they are, and recognize when they are going through a rough period of time. Lift them up. So often I hear people say we only hear from the boss when we mess up. I have been fortunate to have a long history of supervisors who do care about my struggles as long as I am willing to let them in and understand. It makes a difference.

Take advantage of the Critical Incident Stress Management (CISM) program. If you're not familiar with this, there's training out there. Execute the CISM debriefings from the viewpoint of the people in the field. Don't generalize their emotions because everybody in that room is going to be in a different place according to their experience. Identify the providers trying to be strong so as not to look weak. Follow up with everybody the next day, the next week, the next month. When the anniversary approaches, watch them. Is their head in the game or are they reliving all the emotions they've suppressed for the last year?

Above all, be kind to each other. We all know that the worst call of our career is only a phone call away. Check on each other. Support each other. It's easy to be petty. It's godly to love. Carry that phone number for crisis intervention in your wallet. When you see that something is wrong pull it out and reassure them you care.

The Army taught us to use our ACE card. If you serve in the military, you know the best way to pass the time is by playing cards. At least it was before social media and smartphones. They taught us if we are worried about somebody, pull the ACE card.

<u>A</u>sk, flat out, are you going to hurt yourself?

<u>C</u>are for the person. Sit with them and let them get it out in the open where their head is at.

<u>E</u>scort them to a safe place.

We see it all the time in the movies. A soldier is shot. They're lying out in the open. The squad or platoon sees that if they leave him in that position he is going to die. They get to him and throw on a tourniquet to stop the bleeding. Then they drag him off to a safe place to evaluate how to fix him. It's the same thing. It's just that in this case the war is on the inside. And the casualties are piling up.

Escort them to somebody with a higher ability to help. Is there an employee assistance program where you work? Is there a designated crisis worker team? Can you sit down with somebody in the emergency department after the patient is turned over to a higher level of care? Can you invite them to church to offer a change of scenery? Do you have chaplains you can call to counsel

the individual? If none of these options are feasible, why not?

Get to know your coworkers. What do they enjoy? What is

their family like? Are they themselves religious? Maybe they have

a different fashion than you. Maybe they eat different things based

on religious or dietary or cultural background. It doesn't matter.

I'm not telling you to become their roommate. I'm only asking

that you care and let them know you care because you, not your

management, have the ability to recognize a change in them.

If you've read this book and want more information about

God and His promises and what He can and will do for you, that's

amazing. My first recommendation is going to be to find out more.

In the palm of your hand is a device that can connect you to so

much. Find out what churches are close to where you live. Get on

social media to see if they have an account where they post videos.

Try them on like you try on a new pair of shoes or an outfit.

Maybe it looks good, but it isn't your fit. That's fine. Try another one. I had a church my parents took me to. I tried a church that a friend attended. I went to church on Sunday in basic training to get out of the work of polishing our barracks. I attended so many funerals in my life that brought me into a variety of different churches. I went to a church with Tommy that we could take the ambulance to and nobody scoffed at us if our pager activated for a call. Maggie and her mom took us to church. Finally, we found the one that spoke to us. We found a home, a community of people [our age] who believe as we believe and understand that when the kids aren't behaving in public, there's a chance you won't be as good a reflection of Jesus as you are trying to be. But you're already forgiven. Find your church. Tell somebody you want to learn more. So many people will be willing to sit down and talk to you and answer your questions.

Finally, friends, I ask you this. Share this book with somebody. I said early on that my experience may be vastly different than many, but it also may be along the lines of somebody's struggle you aren't aware of. My hope for this book is that through its pages and through God's wisdom we can prevent

even one more soul lost to suicide, domestic violence, or poor self-

control leading to imprisonment. He knows your name. He knows

your struggles. He loves you regardless. God loves you, and so do

I.

"I rejoiced in the Lord greatly that now at length you have

revived your concern for me. You were indeed concerned for me,

but you had no opportunity. Not that I am speaking of being in

need, for I have learned in whatever situation I am to be content. I

know how to be brought low, and I know how to abound. In any

and every circumstance, I have learned the secret of facing plenty

and hunger, abundance and need. I can do all things through Christ

who strengthens me."--Philippians 4:10-13

<u>Acknowledgments</u>

First, I would like to thank the colleagues I've worked with or volunteered with over the past 20 years. You all helped me write my story by going through it all with me, whether you knew it or not.

To my church: You have been my biggest cheerleaders in writing this book. You have shown me God like I have never seen before. I am grateful for the work God is doing in our life and even more so that we have this community to be His conduit for us.

And to my wife: I love you more today than I ever have before. You have been God's biggest blessing in my life. You and I have powered through so much, and we did it all together. My life is complete because you are in it. We built a family and a life together that I would not trade for anything in the world. I know that no matter where life takes us, we'll be just fine because we have each other. My love for you has never faltered; it's only gotten stronger. I look forward to sharing this book with our children and one day grandchildren to show them what it is to love like your life depends on it. Babe, I love you so much. I'll love you forever until the day I die, and it still won't be long enough.

www.ingramcontent.com/pod-product-compliance
Lightning Source LLC
Chambersburg PA
CBHW070335220526
45467CB00001B/139